Bedroom Games

Bedroom Games

STRIPTEASES, SEDUCTIONS, AND OTHER SURPRISES TO KEEP YOUR PARTNER COMING BACK FOR MORE

MARY TAYLOR

THREE RIVERS PRESS
NEW YORK

Published by Three Rivers Press, New York, New York.
Member of the Crown Publishing Group, a division of
Random House, Inc.

www.randomhouse.com

THREE RIVERS PRESS and the Tugboat design are registered trademarks of Random House, Inc.

Printed in the United States of America

DESIGN BY ELINA D. NUDELMAN

Library of Congress Cataloging-in-Publication Data is available upon request.

ISBN 0-609-80974-1

10 9 8 7 6 5 4 3 2 1

First Edition

To my grandmother, Mamma Genia,
whose chicken soup first taught me
the joys of stirring the pot

Acknowledgments

It has been a long road for me from naive schoolgirl, to single mom, to exotic dancer, and finally to seduction instructor and author. The people I have met on the journey have been, to say the least, interesting. You will meet many of them in this book. There is, however, another group of people not mentioned in this book whose support and guidance helped me choose the direction to take each time I reached those inevitable forks in the road. Sometimes they helped me see that there was a route to take when I could only see obstacles in my path. For them I offer these humble acknowledgments.

My parents, Antonio and Teresa, have given me their love and support throughout my entire life, regardless of my choices. Without them, I would not have had the courage to choose the path that ultimately led to this book. Their helpful contributions have recently extended to a very reasonable rent for the basement apartment in their house (in which this book was written) and my mother's homemade pasta, which was brought to me when I was too engrossed in work to think about eating properly.

Mary Shaver is a magical person who entered my

life as my eighth grade teacher. Her love and wisdom have been an inspiration to me, and the confidence she gave to me has remained throughout my entire life. So has her friendship and guidance.

My son, Jason, whose stable presence and unconditional love have supported me for thirty years now, first gave me the strength to believe I could change my life for the better. I extend my love along with my gratitude.

Permit me the indulgence to thank my beautiful German shepherd, Keetah. Without her big brown eyes and persistent begging I would never have taken those much-needed walks (sometimes at one A.M.) and had a chance to stop and smell the roses or gaze at the stars—essential diversions if one is to sustain the energy needed to complete a book.

I give my heartfelt thanks to my friend Sylvie, a strong and beautiful woman in every way. By asking for my help, she showed me how to help myself while giving women something I didn't know I had to give.

Thanks to my friend, mentor, and literary agent, Ken Atchity, who inspired me and prodded me to get off my ass and actually write this book. He believed I could do it long before I did.

Ken's considerable efforts led me to Three Rivers Press and the highly capable editorial skills and enthusiastic support of Carrie Thornton. She holds the distinction of being the first person to try the seductive moves I describe in this book without benefit of my personal instruction or video. If you, the reader, can get through these moves without injury and with a smile on your face, it is becuase she has gone before you.

A book is about many things—hopes, dreams, information, enlightenment, entertainment—but ultimately it must be about words. In my own humble way with words, I wish to thank my editor and, by now, close friend, Howard Linscott. He has taken my ideas and my passion and given them form and shape. With two years of his life heavily invested in this project, he ran the considerable risk of becoming bored and frustrated, not only with me, but with the subject of stripping and seduction. I am happy to report that neither has occurred.

Finally, thanks to my many friends and cheerleaders, too numerous to list, whose stories and ideas have found their ways onto these pages. This includes the many dancers I have met throughout the years and the courageous ones that moved on to new careers, as well as all the men who have cheered me on during my years as an entertainer. But my deepest gratitude goes to the thousands of women who have taken my classes. You have touched my heart. You are the brave ones for taking action!

Contents

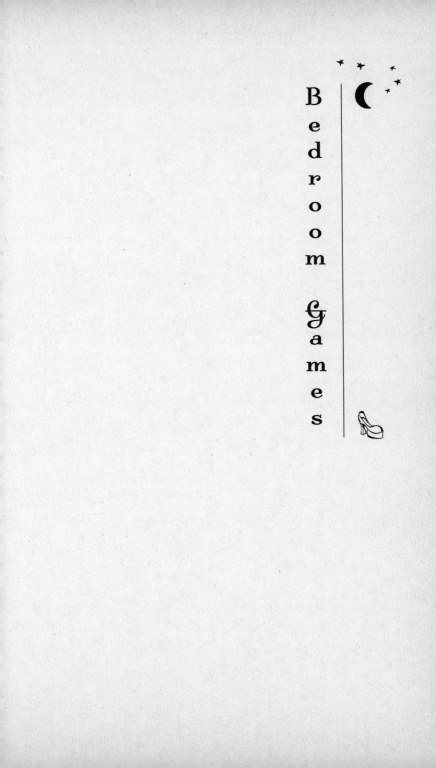

Bedroom Games

Every Woman's Fantasy

I believe that deep down, every
woman thinks of what it would be like to
perform an erotic striptease. Her fantasy
involves slowly and seductively removing
her clothes for an audience of at least one
enthusiastic, highly appreciative man.
Imagine yourself in this scene:

You call your loverboy, and his manner
on the phone and his relaxed tone of voice
indicate a frisky and receptive mood.
After days of teasing and prepping him
for a "big night" without
letting the secret out of the
bag, you let it slip that you

have a special surprise planned for this evening. You hang up the phone and dive into the preparations. Your vision for this evening is now turned into action. The pages you've read in all those trashy romance novels or the scenes you've seen in those sexy movies are jumping out at you as you move the coffee table out of the way. First you remove the lightbulbs from their sockets and replace them with bulbs that emit a subtle blue glow. Melted stubs of wax are replaced with scented candles. A slow, seductive CD is cued up to your favorite song. Next comes the food for your feast. You set the table for the kill, with seduction foods like chocolate and fruit, oysters and caviar. Satisfied with your work so far, you slip beneath the foam of a hot bath and begin to relax.

The question of what to wear poses no problem as you sashay up to the closet and dig out your hidden treasure. The French maid's outfit you picked out last week is ready to work its magic. The black stockings have seams running down the back and little satin bows at the start of your ankles. Your black bra and panties are a matching set. With only half the fabric of a real maid's outfit, this cute little number has short sleeves and laces up in front down to the waist. Below the waist, the skirt flares out to stop just below the bottom of your cheeks. As you would expect, the apron is white with frilly trim all the way around, and wraps around the back to tie into a big bow. Oh, I almost forgot: The ensemble is set off by cute little frilly gloves with the fingers cut out and a matching white-lace cap that sits just back on your head.

It's time. At seven o'clock he walks in the door and into your homemade den of seduction. You meet him at the door dressed as his personal maid—a greeting any man would find hard to resist. Your little white frilly apron points to your garter belt as it peeks out of the bottom of your dress. His eyes trace the seams in your stockings all the way down to the four-inch heels of your patent-leather pumps. His eyes light up as the smile on your face gives him only a glimpse of what lies ahead for the evening.

"Would you like a cocktail, monsieur?" you ask with a Lolita-like tone in your voice. He gulps as your finger beckons him to follow you into the living room. You lead him by the tie and then, placing your hands on his shoulders, push him into the large, overstuffed chair. Little does he know how hard you have been practicing for the last two weeks.

You slither slowly into the kitchen, giving him an enticing view of your tush. You come back with a tray of goodies and gently place the hors d'oeuvres in his mouth. As you lick your lips, you move away with a deadly wiggle. He watches you pour a drink with long, sweeping motions. The cold liquid drips into the glass. Standing between his legs, you place the glass to his lips, spilling a small drop down his chin. Your tongue licks his chin clean. You whisper an apology for making him "a little wet." When he tries to fondle you, you push his hands away and put them by his side.

It's time to turn on the stereo. You take your time; every movement is like foreplay. Nothing will be rushed tonight. The music starts and so do you. Now it's time to peel and play!

Standing in front of him, you ask in a seductive voice, "Is there anything else I can do for you, monsieur?" You strut around in front of him, playfully fingering your apron. All the time, the music is playing and you are dancing. Slowly you take the apron strings in your fingers and begin to untie them. Carefully moving the apron back and forth, you tease him with a glimpse of your panties under your short skirt. Then you turn around and toss your apron with attitude, hitting him in the face. You undo the laces on the front of your dress one at a time as your body moves to the music. You wiggle out of your dress, pulling it off your shoulders and dropping it to the floor. Pointing your toes, you kick the dress out of the way, because now it's time to get closer.

He has suffered enough—almost. You've saved the big move you have been practicing. Crouching in front of him as he sits in the chair, you trace a line up his thighs with your fingers, and then on up to his chest until you are in a standing position with your arms on his shoulders. With your body straight, you lean forward until your breasts lightly brush his face. Slowly, gracefully, seductively, you slide down the length of his body, sliding your breasts over every inch of him until you stop gently on the floor at his feet. He's squirming in his chair and you push his frantic hands away. Oh, he wants you all right.

But not yet—it's time for him to take a few things off, too. That tie has got to go. Taking the tip of it in your mouth, you growl and shake your head around like a hungry animal. You use the tie to spank yourself gently. Undoing each of his shirt buttons, you uncover his bare chest and give his erect nipple a little lick, again asking, "Can I get you anything else, monsieur?" Without listening for his answer, you prove it's *your* show by placing your foot on his thigh. You unclip your garter and roll your stockings down one leg at a time. You straddle his struggling form and begin kissing his neck and whispering in his ear.

You repeat this Front Slide (a move you'll learn in detail later) and find yourself between his legs, facing his crotch. With a soft touch to feel his erection, you lie down on your back and carefully slip your heels out of your shoes and flip them one by one over your head and across the room. You play with your breasts, savoring the moment before removing your bra. As you straddle him once again, he needs no coaxing to taste your fabulous breasts. Only for a moment, though, because you still have one more song to dance to before you let the "master" have his way. In actuality, of course, you are the one having *your way*. He is putty in your hands for the rest of the evening—maybe longer! You have created the illusion in his overheated brain (and elsewhere) that you are his maidservant for the night.

Does that sound like what you have been imagining? "Noooo," you say to yourself. "I'm a *good girl*. I've been brought up properly to know right from wrong and could never have such thoughts."

Think again, sister!

I believe it is perfectly normal, even healthy, to entertain such a fantasy. All women want more than anything else to be loved and appreciated. Many women are lucky enough to achieve the love they seek from close, long-term relationships, one man at a time. Others, including entertainers but most notably strippers, get the love and admiration they crave in strong but short-term doses from men they barely know. Are these the "bad girls"?

The point to remember is that both the "bad girl" and the "good girl" are motivated by the same healthy, perfectly normal drive for love and admiration. From the time we are little girls through our teenage years and into adulthood—and in fact for our whole lives— women get the message that the good girl is the only girl to be. Many of us live in denial of the bad girl inside of us and suppress her fantasies. I believe that the mature, well-balanced female personality will integrate both these sides, good and bad, and get just what she wants out of her relationship.

Until six years ago, my "bad girl" was the one who brought home the bacon. For two decades I earned a good living as a stripper, dancing in clubs across the country. During that time I saw the stripping industry change as it never had before. In the mid 1970s when I started dancing, the stars of the business and the chief moneymakers for the clubs were the feature dancers. Exotic dancers in the true sense of the word, they had costumes and routines to match their exotic names. The rich heritage of burlesque was still in evidence when women like Busty Monroe and Chesty Morgan were on-stage. The men in the audience understood that it was about fun as well as sex, and enjoyed an atmosphere that was bawdy but not tawdry. G-strings remained on and there was no touching allowed. Dancers were seen only onstage where they belonged—above the crowd.

From Stage Play to Foreplay

By the 1990s "exotic dancing" had changed from stage play to little more than foreplay. A few feature dancers remained, and all dancers were expected to do some sort of show onstage, but by the 1990s the industry was dominated first by table dancing, and later by lap dancing. Table dancers would carry their platforms with them, plunk them in front of a patron, and dance inches from his face. A lap dance consists of wriggling and squirming on a patron's lap. Fondling is discouraged sporadically, if at all. In most jurisdictions, total nudity is now permitted by law. Rather than working as contracted professional entertainers the way strippers had in the past, table and lap dancers solicited openly for their business on the floor of the club, remitting fees or a percentage of their take to the club owners. Does this sound a lot like another profession to you? It does to me, too.

This change was accomplished largely due to the scheming of strip-club owners, using classic labor-busting techniques. Typically, club owners would bring in inexperienced young girls from a nearby area, or even more successfully, from a foreign, usually Third World country, who were willing to table- or lap-dance and pay a percentage of their earnings to the owner.

These girls had little more than their willingness to recommend them; they generally lacked any qualifications or experience as dancers or entertainers. The local strippers were told to do table and lap dancing in addition to their stage acts, or leave. Whenever the issue attracted public attention, club owners successfully hid under a cloak of free expression or some similar rationalization. The media was often distracted by the morality inherent in the topic, missing its true character as a labor issue.

I love classic burlesque—the corny jokes and suggestive skits from the comedians, the elaborate costumes and routines of the dancers. To me this is an adults-only playground: a chance to peel and play, with no worry about the kids. It's that burlesque spirit that got me into the business of stripping. For years I enjoyed the same thrill that motivates any entertainer who works before a live audience. When it stops being fun, I used to say, I want to get out. Well, it stopped being fun. The lifestyle had me hooked, though, and it took me a few years to realize the fun was gone. I was forced to travel more and more, and further and further, if I wanted to work as a feature dancer on the increasingly rare feature stages. Lap dancing and table dancing were hard to endure. So I quit.

Twenty years as a stripper can teach you a lot about

STRIPPER VS. EXOTIC DANCER— WHAT'S THE DIFFERENCE?

IN THE OLD DAYS WHEN STRIPPING WAS TRULY EXOTIC DANCING, THE WOMEN CALLED THEMSELVES STRIPPERS. NOW THAT THE BUSINESS INVOLVES LITTLE MORE THAN STRIPPING YOUR CLOTHES OFF, THE WOMEN WHO DO IT LIKE TO REFER TO THEMSELVES AS EXOTIC DANCERS.

life, but it doesn't give you many skills that can easily be transferred to a nine-to-five labor market. Twenty years of hiding what you do for a living from your family and people in the "normal" world leaves its psychological scars as well.

When I quit dancing, I didn't think I was smart enough, or good enough, or good-looking enough to do anything else. I hid my feelings, working menial jobs in the quest for a "normal" life. Eventually, on occasion, I was comfortable enough to mention my past career to women I encountered. Their reactions came as a surprise. Rather than dismiss me or move on to a more familiar topic, as I expected they would, they'd ask me, with eyes opened wide, for more details. "Weren't you scared when you went up there?" "What was it like to dance onstage and take your clothes off, sometimes in front of hundreds of men?" "Where were some of the places you traveled, and what were the clubs like?" "What sorts of men go to strip clubs?"

A Stripped-Down Curriculum

Most of their questions centered on my actual stage performances, the moves I made, what I wore, and the songs I danced to. At the end of each of these gab sessions the same thing would happen: The women would ask me to teach them how to do some of my seductive moves so they could surprise their partners on birthdays, for anniversaries, or just *because*.

At first I shrugged off their requests. I didn't want to dwell on my past. But it soon became apparent that their interest was genuine, and that these women really did want to learn how to do this at home. This seemed very odd to me. When I was dancing for a living, the last thing I ever wanted to do was go home and strip for my guy! Everybody I associated with either stripped for a living, like me, or had seen it often enough to be disinterested. But this subject was truly new to the women I was meeting now, and they had no idea where to start.

Here was a chance for me to put my heart and soul into a new career, and use the experience gained during twenty years of my life for a worthwhile purpose. A quick check revealed that there were few books or instructional videos for anyone who wanted to learn how to strip; moreover, the material I found was dated, and aimed solely at the professional stripper. I had hardly been a student in my life, however, let alone a teacher, and I wasn't sure how to put together a course on stripping no matter how much I knew my subject.

Monique is one of those people who come into your life for a reason. Tall and beautiful, Monique taught French to adults, and spoke with a charming French-Canadian accent. She became my first student. Monique wanted to learn the moves of a professional stripper. How would I teach her? Everything I did onstage had become second nature to me, and it would require a lot of conscious analytical thought on my part before I could explain it to others. Before I could tell her how to move, I needed to know what Monique would be wearing, what music she would be dancing to, and the character she planned to portray. That's when I realized that my course of instruction wasn't going to be only about the moves.

Drawing heavily upon Monique's experience as a teacher, we created the core of the "curriculum" I have been teaching for the past four years. I thought back to the questions women had been asking me and decided I would have to address two central issues before I could begin to teach the techniques of stripping. Those issues were fear and self-acceptance.

We all are at least a little fearful before we start something new. Nothing can compare to taking your clothes off in front of others as a fear generator. After all, isn't that literally every woman's worst nightmare? And stripping isn't the sort of activity where you can "learn the trade" by apprenticing or by watching others, so I was sure this would be *very* new to all the women I would be teaching.

Women in our culture are bombarded daily with images of idealized female types. Who can possibly hope to compare to Nicole Kidman or Britney Spears? Even someone like Monique, who is a beautiful woman, seemed to be insecure about her appearance. I knew I would have to address this almost universal insecurity before my students would have the confidence to attempt the actual stripteasing moves.

This book will follow the order and content of my "Peel and Play" workshops. After offering my thoughts on overcoming fear and accepting ourselves the way we are (Chapters 3 and 4), I talk about communication. Think of this as intelligence gathering. Learning more about your own and your partner's fantasies can only help make your seductions more erotic and memorable. Chapters 6 and 7 will help you choose a role and costume for your evening. (Suddenly it's Halloween, with a bigger treat in store than candy!) Setting the stage for your evening of seduction will take considerable planning, even if you aren't keeping your plans a secret from your partner. Chapter 8 tells you how to create a memorable scenario. Most of all, the women who attend my "Peel and Play" workshops enjoy learning to shake their booties like the pros. Chapter 9 outlines in detail some basic moves that pros use, and suggests a basic sample routine. Chapters 10 and 11 describe some additional moves for those who want to take it as far as they can go. If "as far as you can go" means doing your own strip-a-gram, then Chapter 12 is for you!

Bob's Life—Every Man's Fantasy

After my first experience teaching, I knew I needed personal assistance in the classroom. Like those well-established Tupperware parties we've all been to, my first workshop took place in a private home as a small gathering of friends. The moves I taught were borrowed largely from the routines of lap dancers, with a few moves from the "floor shows" of stage dancers thrown in. Here is what I had envisioned for my first workshop: Much like the table and lap dances the "pros" did in clubs, the dance my students would learn took place immediately in front, and right on the laps of, their partners, who would be sitting. To demonstrate the moves, I therefore used an empty chair kindly provided by my hostess. This was less than satisfactory, so to make the motions more clear, I would demonstrate a move on someone in the class. Needless to say, this did not help anyone relax!

Bob came to the rescue and volunteered to be a partner substitute, surely every man's private fantasy. But Bob isn't like other men. Bob is a commercial store dummy, who's now been rescued from a life of modeling men's clothing in a shop window. He can be posed in any position and, starting in my second workshop, he sits through all the giggles and awkward first moves of my students without complaint. Soft on the outside but always stiff inside (foam rubber over flexible-rod construction), quiet and well dressed—not to mention always available—he is the ideal man according to some of my students. Bob wears his Italian suit at all times and travels to my workshops sitting next to me in my two-seater Mercedes convertible. It can be hard on a woman's ego, though; Bob gets more friendly smiles and waves when we travel than I do!

2

After I share with my students my story of how I came to teach this subject and why, I often go around the room and everyone gets a chance to reply to the question "What are you doing here?" or "Why did you take this workshop?" In your case, dear reader, I might ask you, "Why did you buy this book?"

The answers I get from the women attending my workshops fall into six categories.

Which one applies to you?

I. YOU HAVE BEEN IN A RELATIONSHIP FOR A LONG TIME AND THINGS ARE GETTING A LITTLE DULL.

You've been fantasizing about what it was like in the beginning of your relationship when things were fresh and new and exciting and you used to make love in places besides the bed. . . . What happened? Your children may be grown and out of the house, and you find yourself alone with someone you don't have much in common with anymore. You still get along, but are afraid to get truly romantic because you don't know what kind of reaction you will get. You want to rekindle the embers of your passion into a roaring blaze!

2. YOU ARE IN AN EXCITING, NEW, OPEN RELATIONSHIP AND YOU ARE EXPERIMENTING WITH EACH OTHER.

So far you've been enjoying a fun and playful sexual relationship. You want that playtime feeling to continue and improve. You want to reach the highest levels of sensuality you have ever experienced.

3. YOU ARE SINGLE AND WANT TO PREPARE FOR ANY FUTURE RELATIONSHIPS.

You haven't yet attempted a long-term relationship, but you want any new lover to know you are hot! You think that if you can learn to strip, you can do anything. Maybe you're looking for a little ego and confidence boost.

4. YOUR GIRLFRIEND DRAGGED YOU TO THE WORKSHOP.

Your best friend thought it would be fun, so she used you as an excuse. Perhaps she was too chicken to admit she was dying to find out what really happens at a workshop called "Peel and Play." For those of you standing in a bookstore flipping through this book, maybe your girlfriend suggested you buy it, check it out, and pass it around among your friends. Bad idea. All of you will need your own personal copy so you can highlight your favorite parts and use it for your daily practice sessions!

5. YOU ARE DOING RESEARCH FOR A NOVEL OR SHORT STORY.

Believe it or not, I hear this regularly. Every other workshop I do, a woman gives research as her reason for being there. If only half of them are telling the truth, there must be a lot of novels with hot seduction or stripping scenes out there on the bookshelves. Maybe you'll want to do a little research of your own by the time you finish this book.

6. IT BEATS LOOKING AT TUPPERWARE.

No doubt this is true for just about everyone. I'll admit it. I used to sell Tupperware when I first quit dancing, and saw the same cross-section of women at Tupperware parties that I see now. Somehow, helping women keep their leftovers fresh isn't as fun or as satisfying as keeping their sex lives fresh.

All these reasons are good reasons for taking one of my workshops or, in your case, buying this book. People doing so for reasons 4 through 6 are going to get more than they expected, even if they still have to throw out a few leftovers.

So . . . why *do* you want to do this?

With four years of teaching behind me, I have learned that the true reasons for taking my "Peel and Play" workshops run deeper than the six motives given above. As much as I would like to, I know that I am not turning this nation, woman by woman, into a land of secret seductresses. No, most of the women I see have reasons that are more personal, more internal. Perhaps you've always wanted to learn what strippers know because:

7. YOU FEEL THAT DEEP DOWN INSIDE SOMEWHERE, SOMETHING IS SMOLDERING.

You suspect this something is an unexplored sensual side of yourself. You want to know what it feels like to express your sensuality more openly, more freely. You suspect that getting in touch with your inner passions will have beneficial effects that spill over into other aspects of your life.

I strongly suspect this is the true reason most women end up in my workshops. Being a mother, wife, executive, employee, daughter, student—each of these roles alone is very demanding of our time and energy. When putting them together in some combination, as we all must do, we can easily lose track of our core being. The first thing that seems to go is our sensuality. In a life full of doing things for others, we've lost the bad girl inside, the bad girl who knows exactly what she wants and how she is going to get it. Somehow we can all sense the loss, even if we can't put our finger on it.

As I watch the women in my workshops interact, I have gradually come to understand that there is often yet another motive for learning the arts of seduction— one that involves curiosity. I believe the women in my workshops are, to borrow a term from Wall Street, "benchmarking" their romantic lives. All the "opening up" and frank talk as we discuss our fears, complaints,

Benchmarking is a performance-based standard that rejoices in attaching numbers to things. But what would the quantifiable standards of a good romance be? One proposal: total duration (in minutes) of sexual encounters per week divided by number of sexual encounters plus total duration of skin-to-skin contact per day (in minutes) times the number of naughty words spoken per day (benchmark mean estimated at 138). Or should we be measuring the rate and increase in heartbeat and blood pressure during personal encounters? Not to mention blood flow to vital organs. Medical science, Arthur Andersen—someone please help.

and hopes is an opportunity to draw the same information from others. As much as they want to do better, the women in my workshops are eager to know that, compared to the romance others are (or aren't) getting, they are doing just fine. I'm sure most of the women taking my workshops conclude that they are. For you, the reader, you still won't know exactly what your neighbors are doing in their love lives when you finish this book, but you'll be willing to bet they aren't having the fun you are!

No doubt your partner approves of your interest in learning to strip, now that he has seen you with this book. Maybe he even bought this book for you. How about that for a clear message? But a word of caution is called for here. Your reasons for doing this should be your own. Any professional working in the field of mental health will tell you that the patient's desire to improve is crucial to his or her success at doing so. No amount of coaxing from loved ones will keep someone in a course of therapy if they haven't decided that they must change. The motivation has to come from within. The same is true for someone embarking on a course in the art of seduction.

One day I got a phone call from a man inquiring about my workshops. He wanted to register his wife. When I asked him why his wife did not call herself, he had no answer for me. I guessed to myself that perhaps she didn't speak English. I gladly gave him as much information as I could and didn't give it any more thought.

My next workshop date came around and all the participants laughed as they shared their reasons for attending. In the course of the discussion some of the women talked about how their partners wanted them to learn how to strip. I often heard this, but I sensed that these women had their own reasons for coming besides pleasing their men. One woman had been very quiet. She seemed frightened when she told me her husband had enrolled her in the workshop. She was suffering from nervousness, I thought, but that would pass as we all got into the fun of choosing our roles, deciding on an outfit, and learning the moves.

As the evening progressed, everyone laughed their way to a good time except this one woman. She never did get comfortable, and only joined in when pushed. The next day, I got a call from a man who complained that his wife had been in my workshop the evening before but had not learned what the course promised. Then the other shoe dropped. He was the guy who had called to enroll his wife, and she was the woman who was so uncomfortable the evening before! I explained in no uncertain terms what I thought about his actions. It was unfair to force this sort of activity on her. Somehow he thought he could send his wife and that in one night of instruction I could transform her into a stripper goddess. Whatever his/her/their problem was, I explained to him, it could best be dealt with by a professional therapist, not by me or in my class.

So, learning to strip for your partner is not a form of therapy. It might work to loosen a few muscles in your hips and it will certainly make you feel better about yourself and maybe just a tad wicked and sexy, but don't use it to fix a broken marriage. In fact, it could make things worse. If you don't get the positive response you expect, you may feel as though you have failed again. Don't do this to yourself. If you have got problems in your relationship, seek out a pro experienced with cases like yours, someone you are comfortable with. Or spend your energy on getting out of an unsatisfactory relationship. Look forward to a future with someone who appreciates you and deserves you, and remember that you are a B.I.T.C.H—Beautiful, Intelligent, Talented, Charming, and Hot!

I can't promise an objective standard against which to measure your romantic encounters, but I can promise you will be getting a chance to view, to borrow another phrase from Wall Street, "Best Practices." Reading this book will give you a chance to sample the best techniques and moves of the women who make seduction their business. How far you want to take it is up to you.

I also hope this book turns out to be more than just a good read. Feel free to set your goals higher than just having fun creating some sexy outfit and learning some dance moves. You may wish to treat this as an opportunity to explore your sensuality. This can be as simple as appreciating the erotic power of touch. I was reminded recently of how uplifting this lesson can be.

One of the basic moves I show the women in my workshops involves fondling or playing with their own breasts. After all, if you don't know how to give yourself pleasure in this way, how can you expect him to know? Well, one woman felt too uncomfortable to do this in front of her friends. I doubt that she had ever done this in private, either. But eventually, after watching the other women having fun, she tried a few tentative strokes. The message hit home fast. By the end of the workshop she was moving 'em around like the best strippers I have seen. It changed her whole attitude and the way she approached the more difficult dance moves.

This change in attitude, increase in confidence, or loss of fear—whatever you want to call it—is the main thing women bring home from my workshops and the main thing you should get from this book. If taking off your clothes and exposing your sensual core to someone else is the scariest thing you can imagine doing and you still do it, what is there left to fear? What is there you cannot accomplish? The confidence you gain by executing your own seduction scene will spill over into other areas of your life. Besides the obvious benefit of being more self-expressed in a more open relationship, your new self-confidence will help you do those things you've been wishing you could do for so long, such as quitting an unfulfilling job to start a business of your own, or speaking with assurance in front of others. One woman I taught told me that it gave her the confidence she needed to tackle the redecoration of her house! I know what courage that takes; I tried it myself once, too.

Up and Off on the Roof

One very fortunate workshop I taught last year got the results they hoped for, and a little more, much sooner than they ever expected. I'm often called to do presentations at bridal showers. The hostesses of these events want them to be like female versions of the stag parties their fiancés are having—a sort of final flinging off of the single life. So it's either hire me or a male stripper to zip things up. On this occasion, Brenda had another surprise in store for her friends besides me and my tutorial. Her bridal shower would be on the rooftop terrace of her ten-story apartment building. Events were to start early Friday night so that everyone could head out to a nightclub afterward to show off the brand-new sexy moves they had learned.

Ten flights of stairs carrying a dummy whose head keeps banging against the walls is not my idea of a great date, but the setting proved to be worth it. The rooftop terrace was attractively lit, and the table set with cocktails and ice. A tray of sushi was provided. The mother of the bride, two of her friends, and the bridesmaids sat with Brenda in a semicircle nervously anticipating the tips I would provide for them. The trip upstairs had been tough on Bob, so I straightened out his shirt and tucked it into his pants. He sat off to the side waiting for his chance to spring into inaction.

Soon after I began speaking, one of the women in our party noticed that a light had been flashing rhythmically on and off in the high-rise building across the way. Several men were waving from the balcony and holding something up for us to see. It was a phone number. Realizing they were trying to get our attention, we stopped what we were doing. One of the girls got out her cell phone and called the number. It turns out this was a group of guys just relaxing and having a few drinks on a Friday night before getting ready to go out. It must have been the first time they had seen eight beautiful women on a rooftop with a dummy.

When they asked what we were doing, Brenda told them we were learning how to strip for our lovers, and that I was the presiding expert. The guys could barely believe their good fortune. They were like a bunch of children who just got news that school had been canceled. They were told to keep their eyes glued to the terrace in a half hour for the part of the workshop where we learned to do some actual stripping moves. They patiently waited on their eighteenth-floor balcony with hangdog looks on their faces.

When we got to the moves, the boys could no longer stand still. They found some sort of floodlight and began beaming it in our direction. Christmas minilights swayed back and forth, and the apartment interior lights were flicked on and off. From where we stood, their apartment looked like a theater stage. Everyone laughed. A lot of "creative juices" were flowing from these guys on the eighteenth floor.

By this point we had come to the section of the workshop where I teach my students one by one how to "put their boobs on Bob." Even the mother of the bride and her sixtyish friends were having a ball trying the moves. By now we could see that we were being watched from another location as well. Three stories below where the light show was going on, three men were watching from their apartment window. They turned their lights as bright as they would go, and two of them started to dance for us. The third stripped down to his underwear to show his appreciation.

The guys in the first group soon called us back. When we were nearly done with our workshop, the girls decided to allow the guys to join us on the terrace. Within seven minutes, there were six guys at the bridal shower thanking me for all my assistance and praising the girls for their sensual skills. But it soon became apparent that these guys wanted more than just to join us in the merriment; they wanted pointers, too! So I sat the girls down and had the guys pay back the favor by doing some moves for the ladies. One of them showed an exceptional degree of natural ability. He was kept very busy. Some women hire male strippers for titillation. Ours were unplanned *and* free!

Overcoming Fear

According to Jerry Seinfeld, **3**
public speaking outpolls death as a cause
of fear. That means, he concludes, that
most people would rather be the guy
in the coffin than the guy doing the
eulogy.

As strong as the fear of public speaking
is, I believe there is another fear that equals
it in intensity. This fear is the legendary
theme in our worst nightmares. It is the fear
of being naked in front of an audience.
Even if the audience is only
the man you love, the fear is
real. Obviously, this fear must

be acknowledged before we can begin to learn to strip for our partners.

Good girl or bad girl, we all have little fears that keep us from doing things. I don't mean fears of external things or circumstances, like the fear of flying or closed-in spaces. I mean the fear that kicks in when we are uncertain how we are going to be received by others. After all, as human beings, we all need the love or approval of those around us in order to function. Think of how many of our fears are actually based on this need, and think of the reasons we all create to rationalize them. Do we avoid that dance class because we are out of shape and afraid of the bulges that might show under our Danskin, or because we're afraid of looking foolishly uncoordinated?

Because you have bought this book, you have already taken the first tentative step toward overcoming your fear of stripping for your partner. Good for you. But this is no little fear to deal with, I can hear you thinking, and your brain is busy manufacturing rationalizations. I've heard them all from the women in my workshops. See how convincing they seem (or don't seem) when written down. Have a laugh and then get over it. Here then are the ten reasons I hear most often for not learning how to seduce your partner:

I. MY PARTNER WILL LAUGH AT ME.

Laughter in this case is a sign of nervousness. Yes, *he* might be nervous, too! But this will pass quickly. When men get aroused, they can hold no other thoughts in their minds. Your partner will be thinking only of what he sees and how he is responding to it. If he could hold another thought in his mind at a time like this, he might take a moment to reflect on how you went to so much effort for him.

2. WHAT IF I CAN'T STOP LAUGHING?

Laughter is a normal sign of nervous tension. Just keep your focus on the task at hand. Your nervousness will pass as you become aroused yourself. When women get aroused, they can hold no other thoughts in their minds. Sound familiar?

3. I MIGHT FALL ON MY BUTT.

Not likely with the techniques you will learn in Chapter 9. In the unlikely event that you do fall, it will be the sexiest fall your partner has ever seen. You may even have to do it again.

4. I AM GOING TO LOOK SILLY IN MY COSTUME.

How do you know that when you haven't seen your-self yet? Instead, you will feel the power of your sexuality like never before. You may decide to do battle with your housework dressed as Zena the Warrior Princess from now on.

5. THE NEIGHBORS WILL FIND OUT.

They might. And boy, will you be popular! Expect to be giving advice and distributing copies of this book to them when you've learned how to seduce your partner like a pro. TV sets will be turning off all over your neighborhood after supper.

6. I DON'T HAVE ANY EXPERIENCE DOING ANYTHING LIKE THIS.

Of course you don't. Only professional strippers do. That's why I wrote this book and that's why you bought it. There are still more than 3 billion women like you on this planet who will have to learn sometime. You've got lots of company, and you're ahead of most of them.

7. I MIGHT HURT MYSELF.

You might hurt yourself at the local gym, too, but you've been promising yourself to go there anyway. Promise to do this—it's more fun. And you're more likely to feel better than hurt yourself.

8. I MIGHT LOOK FOOLISH IN FRONT OF OTHERS.

This is a risk only if you plan to do this with friends. You could practice a little before suggesting to your best gal pals that they join you in this activity. In any event, the women who take my workshops find that they get support from one another, not ridicule.

9. I WON'T BE ABLE TO LEARN TO STRIP IN TIME.

In time for what? Don't put any pressure on yourself, and don't tell him what you are doing until you are ready. (In the meantime, you will have to hide this book from him!) You can practice until the neighbors, who have been watching secretly from next store, beg you to go pro. Ha-ha.

IO. I MIGHT TURN INTO A SUPER-SENSUAL SEX VIXEN OUT OF CONTROL.

That's the chance you and your partner will have to take.

All these fears have one thing in common: They exist only in your mind. No doubt about it, the most frightening thing you can do is to take your clothes off in front of someone. Whether the audience consists of one person or one hundred, the fear is the same. But once you have accomplished this challenging task, you learn that you can accomplish anything. The benefits spill over into the rest of your life. Nothing else will ever seem quite so difficult again. Stripping for your partner is really about stripping for yourself. It's about confidence.

There is no apprenticeship program for strippers. You can't go on the road with a feature dancer and help her with her costumes and props until one day you're ready to step into her shoes and out of her costume. Nor can you be a little bit naked. As with being pregnant, you either are or aren't. So, for every stripper there is a first time. For every stripper there is a big-time story of overcoming fear. Here is mine, and what I learned from it.

There's a First Time for Everything

My friend and I had discussed becoming strippers and finally agreed to see an agent. Lori Lane was an ex–burlesque dancer who was happy to show two kids the ropes. Her office walls were covered with hundreds of pictures of strippers. The place smelled of cigarette smoke and contained little more than a telephone, couch, desk, and chair. Lori preferred to recline on her couch, where she sat playing with her hair and touching her body. Running her hand down her leg, she would play with her skirt, exposing her garter and stockings. I watched in wide-eyed amazement. My mind started working overtime. *My legs are too skinny to wear these things. I have no boobs. My nose is too big. Etc., etc.*

Lori showed us a trick of the trade. Slowly, she unclipped a stocking and rolled it down, pinching it between her toes as she unraveled it inside out. Stretching it to its limit, she played with it and made hand-job motions as she stroked the stocking over and over. She finally released it and shot the stocking through the air, letting it fly like a stone out of a slingshot. I thought to myself, no way can I do that; I must be out of my mind. What am I doing here? But before we left, Lori had us both convinced that two beautiful girls like us could earn four hundred dollars a week. Wow! (This was 1976, when minimum wage for a forty-hour week was $126 where I lived.)

So my friend and I gathered up our best disco clothes, including new scarves, stockings, and platform shoes, stuffed them into suitcases, and loaded them into the back of a Ford Pinto. Our first gig was at a place called the Atherly Arms, an hour and a half outside the city, in a small town where we hoped no one would recognize us. As we pulled into the unpaved parking lot, we tasted fear for the first time. The Atherly Arms (known as the Arms 'n' Legs to the locals) was an old run-down barn of a building. The only semblance of a sign was the word WELCOME painted on the white clapboard siding. Nobody had prepared two big-city girls for this.

We left our bags in the car and walked inside. The lights were up and the stench of the previous night's beer and smoke still permeated the place. The carpet had absorbed countless years of spilled brew without a cleaning. A short little guy was bent over behind the bar clearing out the sinks. The floor creaked as we approached.

"Excuse me, we are the dancers who are supposed to be performing here this week." After a brief but polite introduction, he led us upstairs to our rooms. The stairs were wide and groaned under our weight, and the halls were dark and dingy despite their ten-foot-plus height. The Atherly Arms had originally been a train station with a few rooms upstairs for offices or accommodations for affluent travelers. The only rooms now in use on the second floor were occupied by dancers, the band, and one or two tenants whose status I never could determine. The doors to the rooms were at least eight feet high and opened with big, brass doorknobs.

Our room had a sink, but the toilet was a communal affair down the hall. A wardrobe stood with a book holding up the corner where a leg once had been. The dresser was an antique whose drawers no longer closed due to the effects of a dozen or more coats of paint. An old iron-frame bed with a lumpy-looking mattress was pushed up against one wall. The wallpaper mixed a floral pattern with water stains that originated somewhere under the ceiling tile in the corner. The window had glass in most of its panes, and overlooked the parking lot.

We unloaded our suitcases and prepared to settle in for the week. It was now eleven A.M. and the first show was scheduled for twelve o'clock. We numbed our nerves with a bottle of Scotch borrowed from our host. The Scotch was so harsh that not even the sugar and lemon we mixed with it could improve the taste.

As I got ready for my first dance, I caught my reflection in the faded mirror on the wardrobe door. Was I wearing too much makeup? Would anyone even be looking at my face? I certainly had to think of the clothes I would, or rather wouldn't, be wearing. My dress was made of a slinky black fabric that hung to the mid-calf in a scalloped hem. It was held up by ribbon straps with an Indian print. The same ribbon encircled the dress at the bodice, supporting a row of feathers hanging an inch apart. My earrings were matching feathers. The dress was open in front to my waist but tied together with four black ribbons that left small peepholes between them. You could see my belly button if you knew where to look. Underneath was going to be important, too. I wore a black bra, G-string, and T-bar (a high-waisted thong with clips on either side for easy removal). My legs were bare and the sweat on my feet kept my black patent-leather pumps glued to them. I was told I looked like Cher; maybe I did. I was certainly skinny and had long, straight black hair that reached all the way down my back.

It was 11:55 when the owner came knocking at the door and a grizzly voice hollered, "Show time, ladies. Come on down."

Oh, my God! This was really it! I can't do it, I thought. I think I'm gonna throw up! My friend started to panic, too. Amazingly, it occurred to us that we hadn't really thought about what we were going to do onstage until now. It was too late to turn back. My friend had taken a week off from her job at the bank. We both needed the money.

At 12:05 the same grizzly voice returned to the other side of the door. "Ladies, what's the hold-up? I have a full house down there. These guys have only an hour for lunch. Who's on first?" We had been arguing over this point and I guess he'd caught some of it through the door. "I don't care if you both go on together," he said. So we did just that!

Strutting to hide our fear, we headed over to the ancient jukebox to pick out three songs. We hadn't thought about this until now, either. The manager showed up with three coins and we pushed the buttons for three songs we knew.

The crowd looked like a casting call for *The Man Show* (on Comedy Central) and watched our every move as we headed for the dance floor. As the Bee Gees blasted out "Stayin' Alive," my friend and I started into our best disco-dance moves. Twirling each other around eased our nerves a little and we actually began having fun. The audience of country hicks couldn't believe their good fortune. They were going to see two girls get naked before their very eyes at the same time. This was better than tag-team wrestling!

I improvised. I let a man in the front row help me with the laces on my dress. The crowd loved it. The songs raced by and the clothes came off one piece at a time. If the audience noticed our amateurishness, they didn't let it bother them. We got a standing ovation as we left the stage. My friend gently slapped one souvenir hunter who grabbed for the scarf around her neck.

As we were gathering up our costumes, a dancer

came out and strutted toward the jukebox with a huge smile on her face. She must have seen our show. It was obvious she knew which numbers to push off by heart. Her outfit was fabulous and every movement was that of a pro, or so it looked to us. Unlike everyone else in the room, we had never seen a stripper before!

Back in our room, I did throw up and my friend had a little snooze. By one-thirty it was show time again and this time we tossed a coin. Even though we didn't know what we were doing, we now felt like pros. A standing ovation first time out had hooked the natural-born show-off in each of us. We decided that if we could pull this off, we could do anything!

The rest of the week went by like a breeze. Since then I have learned a valuable lesson about overcoming fear: No one ever stops being afraid; the "fearless" just learn to do what they have to do despite their fear. After that first day, every single Monday morning just before I went onstage at a new club, I got an attack of stage fright. It lessened through the years, but it never disappeared entirely. Backstage I thought I would be sick, but as soon as my first foot hit the floor and I felt the music, I was fine.

When you are afraid to do something, visualize the positive results of your action rather than dwelling on the things that could go wrong. In my case, before I went onstage I thought of the power I felt whenever I danced. Every glance I gave someone, I got eye contact in return. I felt connected to my audience as I entertained them. I thought about the adrenaline high performing gave me, rather than the knot in my stomach.

There are many positive results for you to visualize as you go forward with your plans for seduction. By taking a big step and giving pleasure to someone else, you will be opening yourself up to more pleasure in your own life. Your partner will understand why you are performing your seduction. Who knows what he might do to show his appreciation? More important, you will lose your fear of fear itself. Or, rather, fear will lose its grip on you. Nothing will ever seem quite so frightening again. Make a list of things you haven't done because of small fears. Imagine the improvement in your life once you accomplish these things.

For myself, I think back to Jerry Seinfeld's observations on fear. I have long since overcome my fear of being naked in front of others. More recently I have conquered my fear of speaking in public. I figure the only frontier left to conquer is speaking in public while naked.

Constant Complaints

Like so many other grandmothers 4
before and since, my grandma would check
my height by standing me up against a
doorframe to see if I had grown since her
last visit. By the time I was about eleven
years old, Grandma's concern shifted
to other areas. Discreetly, when no one
else was watching, she would feel my
breasts to see if they had grown. My
embarrassment turned to amazement the
day she presented me with my first bra. It

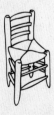 was the tiniest and strangest
piece of clothing I had ever
seen. I barely had nipples, let

alone breasts, and it wasn't clear to me how or why I had to wear this thing. What was she thinking?

My lessons in underwear would continue. I went to a Catholic school, and in those days girls were not allowed to wear pants, except in the winter months, which were very cold where I grew up, when we were permitted to wear pants underneath our dress uniform so long as we removed them when we got to school. This wasn't fun or easy to do. Grandma's thoughtful solution was a pair of thick, green crocheted stockings. The boys would pick on me in the way only eleven-year-old boys can. "Look at that! What NHL team do you think she plays for?" (I guess the boys were still too young to have seen *real* garters and stockings in the Sears catalog.) I was embarrassed and horrified that they might learn what I was hiding under my knee-length tunic dress: My green stockings were held up by the world's tiniest girdle, complete with garters!

My grandmother taught me many things over the years, such as how to make fabulous chicken soup and how to polish a chrome toaster until I could see my reflection. But along with the cooking and cleaning, I absorbed another lesson: I learned to be sensitive about my appearance. Judging by what I hear from the women I meet, I am far from alone.

All women have issues about themselves and their

bodies. Some of these things we can do something about, others we must learn to live with. Whole industries bear witness to women's desire to change whatever can be changed about themselves. Psychoanalysis, exercise classes and videos, hair and cosmetics, and plastic surgery are a few that come to mind.

Understanding what we actually *can* change about ourselves is the first step toward self-acceptance. Any effort we make to change perceived flaws boosts our self-esteem and confidence. Learning to accept the minor imperfections that we can't change is the next step, and a necessary one before we can "take it all off" for our partners.

Complain, Complain

There must be a reason we keep complaining about our looks without doing anything to change them. I confess a secret of mine to the women in my classes. Standing in front of them, I point to my tummy and say, "This is my own biggest personal complaint." In every single class I hear at least two women make comments under their breath like, "Yeah, right, I wish I had a tummy like that." "That is exactly my point," I say. "To you, my tummy is nothing to worry about, but to me, it's a constant source of dissatisfaction." I have twice in the past five years paid for gym memberships and never gone. Why? A tummy is usually something we can change if we really want to.

So I complain about it all the time to my girlfriends and don't do anything about it. "Oh, my God," I say, "I can't wear my little black dress anymore because my tummy is getting so big." Usually my friends respond with something like "Oh, Mary, you look great. I hope I look as good as you when I am your age!" So I straighten myself up, check myself right and left in the mirror, and feel good again. The black dress stays on, and out the door I go.

On those few occasions when I've been in a gym, the first thing the staff ask me is what I would like to work on. So I pull out my well-rehearsed complaint. "I think my tummy needs a little work, and maybe my hips, too." But they don't respond the way my friends do. "Half an hour on the treadmill, twenty minutes on the bike, fifty sit-ups, and when you're done with that, come and see me and I'll give you more things to do." They aren't sucked in by my complaints. A personal trainer won't stroke your ego unless you are accomplishing your goals.

Back home, we sometimes try complaining to our partners. With tired little voices we might say something like, "You know, I'm gaining a little weight lately.

I think I should start jogging or go to the gym." Then we wait for his response. If he's smart (and hasn't heard it too often before), he will say vague, mushy things about how he likes us just the way we are. Some of us try the direct question, such as "Dear, do you think I am too fat?," knowing full well that no man is stupid enough to answer in the affirmative. But if he slips up and we don't hear what we want, the results can be ugly. Once again, we've rigged our conversation so that our minor imperfections get in the way of feeling great about who we are.

So why do we complain about our bodily imperfections and not do anything about them? Because our friends and partners tolerate our attempts to generate sympathy and stroke our egos. And we fall for it every time. It's so much easier than working out. We get lots of juice by complaining to our friends, and nothing but work when we complain to our trainers. My response to this little game is simple: Either get off it . . . or get on it. If you're not going to make the effort or put in the time it takes to change, stop complaining and accept your faults.

Sometimes in my workshops I encourage my students to try an exercise that brings home the same point more personally. I ask them to think about all the things they dislike about their bodies and list them on a piece of paper, omitting their names.

When they are done writing out their lists, I ask them to stand up, choose a partner, and introduce themselves. Once acquainted, they exchange papers, without reading them, and move to the next introduction, repeating the process. When everyone in the class has met, they sit down and open the papers. Nobody has her own list of complaints. Does anyone ever have an empty paper? Never!

Going to the chalkboard, I ask my students to tell me what complaints are written down on the paper in their hands so I can write them down on the board. Every time I do this exercise, I know exactly what the list is going to look like. Big surprise! We all have the same complaints about our bodies. Here they are, in no particular order:

> Cellulite
>
> Nose too big
>
> Lips too thin
>
> Breasts too small
>
> Breasts too large
>
> Stretch marks
>
> Wrinkles
>
> Tummy bulges
>
> Overall size too large
>
> Overall size too small
>
> Too short

Too tall

Hair too fine

Hair too curly

Too fat

Too skinny

Flat butt

No butt

Big butt

Letting Go

The women in my workshops always display some very informative body language when we begin to discuss this topic. They slouch in their chairs with their legs crossed. Their arms are crossed over their breasts. They are so inside themselves you can feel it in the air. Every part of their body is saying, "I don't want to talk about this."

Looking at the list on the board, I ask them, "What are you prepared to do about it? What are you going to do with all that 'stuff' that you have so painfully written down on those tiny pieces of paper?" Then something miraculous happens. One by one, without any prompting on my part, they start to let go of their scraps of paper. Then you can see the beginning of a physical transformation. The last ones to toss their papers are the ones who have the most difficulty letting go and accepting themselves the way they are. When they finally do let go, you can see a marked difference in their demeanor, body language, and movement.

When the complaints of others seem trivial in our eyes, we start to get a glimpse of how foolish our own complaints may be. Marilyn Monroe, still an icon of femininity forty years after her death, certainly wouldn't have contributed anything to our list above, right? Wrong. She worried about the distance between her upper lip and her nose! I can't recall whether she thought it was too small or too large. It hardly matters. That distinctive and sexy smile of hers was designed to hide her flaw from the rest of us. This universal compulsion to find a flaw in one's appearance ensures that something will be found no matter how beautiful a woman really is.

There are other questions we should all be asking ourselves, such as: Who said there is a specific weight that someone has to be? What's in a number, anyway? I tell women to throw their scales away. Get rid of them. Instead, walk up and down a flight of stairs. If you are huffing and puffing, you may want to consider getting into shape simply for health reasons. Do not do it to improve your appearance. If you decide you want to do something about your weight, get your partner to agree to do it with you. Also, positive visualization is a proven

TIP

POST THIS
MESSAGE ON
YOUR
DRESSING
MIRROR:

I AM A
B.I.T.C.H.

BEAUTIFUL,

INTELLIGENT,

TALENTED,

CHARMING,

AND HOT

(OR HORNY,

DEPENDING ON

HOW YOU FEEL)

technique. Put up notes that read, "I am beautiful" or "I am lovable." Remember, you won't need a perfect body in order to strip for someone else, only a body you love.

A note to any men who might be sneaking a peek into this book: Be an active participant in your partner's efforts to improve, not an obstacle. Knock off all the silly, stupid comments about her weight and looks if you are making them! They feel as good to her as nagging over your personal habits feels to you. Create a positive atmosphere in your home. Offer constructive criticism only when asked, and never criticize your partner in front of someone else. Be supportive.

Flash back to grade six. Sitting in front of me was a beautiful girl named Paula. Paula didn't wear thick, green crocheted hose. She was from northern Italy and had blond hair and blue eyes. My parents were from southern Italy, giving me dark hair and eyes like everyone else (or so it seemed). More important, Paula was the only girl in the school with breasts. The boys were so preoccupied with this part of her anatomy that they totally overlooked the size of her nose. I never heard anyone mention it.

So what's my point? Paula probably worries about the size of her nose to this day for all I know. Perhaps she has had a nose job by now, or has gained so much weight that her nose is the last thing on her mind. As this chapter makes clear, no woman seems to be happy with her appearance. But there is another point to be learned here.

All Shapes and Sizes

Boys or men, it doesn't make much difference, we think. Tits, tits, and more tits—that's all they think about when they look at us. And the bigger the better, right? *Wrong*. I want to reassure any of you who might feel light on top that men don't like only large breasts. As one stripper once said, "Men aren't as hung up on breast size as even they think they are." Even the men who go to see strippers are interested in more than just tits, as I was able to prove.

At the height of my dancing days, I didn't look like all the other feature dancers who worked where I wanted to get bookings. They were all gymnasts with bleached blond hair extensions and enormous silicone tits. I couldn't even do the splits, but I worked hard to create a fun show I could share with my audience.

I was able to incorporate my small breasts into my act in several ways. In my Christmas show, I would take off my bra to the tune "I Saw Mommy Kissing Santa Claus" and gently pinch my nipples until they protruded enough to support little candy canes. I would let the guys come over one at a time to claim their Christmas gift. Of course, they had to tip me a dollar to get one. Ho ho ho. Merry Christmas to all, and to all a good night!

Other tricks were possible only because of my 32A size. There was always a guy in the front row puffing on a cigarette. Shortly after removing my bra, I would walk over, pick his cigarette out of the ashtray, pinch my left nipple till it got erect, and balance the lit cigarette on my nipple. Then I would prance around the stage keeping the lit cigarette balanced in its place. Eventually I would return to the cigarette's owner and invite him to retrieve his possession. (Naturally, it never occurs to men to do this with their hands.) I would tease him by moving my breast back and forth in front of his mouth, making it look like he was bobbing for apples. The crowd would roar.

A Big Prize for a Little Lady

The real proof that men willingly accept small boobs came to me in an unexpected way. In the summer of 1983, I got talked into going away for a weekend with a male stripper I was dating named Gary. We planned to go to the country for a camping trip. Gary explained that he and his friend Danny were entering a "beauty" (my word, not his) contest there that would help him make more money as a stripper if he won a title. My girlfriend and I tagged along for the ride, anticipating a fun weekend getaway for four.

When we got there, we found a campground with trailers and campers surrounding a large outdoor stage. Nude men and women were tanning on the rooftops of their campers. Bikini-clad women were running around all over the place. Men were flexing their muscles and strutting around the grounds in their teeny little Speedos. Once we were settled in, we poured ourselves a drink and my friend and I went for a walk to check out the action.

Couples were everywhere. Everyone seemed to be partying and having a good time. We soon learned that the contest wasn't only for men; women were competing in their own category. Our dates immediately suggested that we enter the contest. I was horrified by the idea. I couldn't perform in front of hundreds of people! I had never danced in front of a crowd this large, and there were lots of women in the audience. I had never even dreamt of winning a stripping contest. After all, I had tiny breasts and I always thought I was too skinny to be a feature act. I was quite content just being me.

But they talked us into it. Okay, what the heck, I'll just do this for the fun of it, I thought. It didn't matter to me whether I won or not. I just put a big, happy smile on my face every time I walked on the stage. I enjoyed preparing for each event and modeling the lingerie the sponsors provided. I especially remember a little fringe black skirt with a black-and-red Hawaiian lei around my neck that covered my breasts. As I danced around on the outdoor stage, my nipples were in clear view of the observers, men and women alike. I was surprised by the support of the women in the audience. This was new to me.

That weekend changed everything. I won the title of Ms. Nude 1983–84 for my state, won the lingerie contest, and made first runner-up in the wet T-shirt contest. I took home ribbons, trophies, five hundred dollars in cash, and a contract to do the cover of a magazine. Not bad for someone with no tits and a lot of attitude! My pal was first runner-up for the Ms. Nude title, and her date won the title of Mr. Nude, a trophy, and cash. My boyfriend had arrived with lots of attitude but not the right kind, so all he got was the thrill of driving home with a car full of happy campers.

The Confidence Factor

During my first ten years dancing with these small breasts, it never occurred to me that men wouldn't like me. And I never lacked for men. Women who are comfortable with their appearance will attract men because of their confident attitude, regardless of their breast size.

Have you ever noticed how when you start seeing someone regularly men come out of the woodwork to call you? Where were they when you were stuck at home in your ratty old bathrobe watching *Days of Our Lives* and eating Kit Kat bars cut into dainty bite-sized morsels? This is the confidence factor. Perhaps confidence stimulates those invisible pheromones that attract men without them knowing. Maybe men need to see another man with you to appreciate your "market value." Who knows, but I believe this phenomenon to be real.

A male friend of mine confesses that he is amazed when the women he knows tells him what their appearance complaints are. If he has noticed anything at all, he would describe their "faults" as a matter of personal preference. For example, even a guy who dates only blondes acknowledges that dark hair looks fine; it's just not his preference. The same applies to breast size, as we learned above.

As for the other personal complaints my friend has heard, he claims not to have noticed these elements at all until the woman mentions them! Maybe that should be a lesson to us all. We should never mention our complaints in front of our men. Have you ever made a comment to someone about having a pimple only to have him or her say they hadn't noticed until you mentioned it? It's the same situation.

Yes, there are insensitive pigs out there who criticize women's looks without mercy. I certainly heard them often enough in bars when they were away from familiar female ears. But even in these conversations I didn't hear them criticizing the looks of women they loved, such as wives, girlfriends, mothers, or daughters. So don't give men any ammunition or the permission to start the criticism.

Can You Recognize a Stripper When You See One?

Before I ever started dancing, a neighbor introduced me to a sweet young woman—a girl, really—named Antonietta. Antonietta could not have been twenty and had a pretty face and big brown eyes. She was short and still had that "baby fat" look about her. One day our conversation turned to the subject of money. I griped about how the eighty-seven dollars a week I was being paid to work in a medical clinic was barely enough to pay the bills and support my young child. Then Antonietta shared her secret. She was earning three hundred dollars a week. I was startled and curious. What on earth could she possibly be doing to make that kind of money at such a young age? (Remember, this was 1976.)

Then she dropped her bomb. Antonietta was a stripper! I was shocked. Nothing in my education or experience had prepared me for this. Back then there were no reality TV shows with sex-related topics or any movies that depicted the personal life or stage show of a stripper in a club. The only image that came to my mind was of a pen I had seen once. It had two pictures of women in black bikinis that mysteriously disappeared when you turned the pen over to write.

But Antonietta certainly didn't look like the images on that pen, with or without the black bikini! Since then I have come to know better. During my twenty years as a stripper, I saw every type of woman imaginable take her clothes off onstage. If you were to pass any of them on the street, you would not think, "Oh, look, there goes a stripper." Most of them looked like your next-door neighbor, your sister, your mother, your aunt, your wife, your girlfriend. Even in the change-room in full costume waiting to go on, these women don't look like strippers. Only when they stand on a stage and the lights are turned up does the transformation begin. It happens as soon as that first foot hits the floor. And then she is ON!

I believe the cartoon image of the exotic dancer is perpetrated by the media and by unscrupulous club owners. Where I danced, the agents and club owners were often so particular about what their girls looked like that they only paid big bucks to "features" who had big blond hair with full extensions. The bigger their boobs, the better. It seemed to me that the small-chested dancers, the brunettes, and the girls of color were there only to provide bodies onstage at all times. But I never got that impression from the men in the audience. They loved variety. A successful professional stripper doesn't have to look like the image on the disappearing pens or in the minds of a few men. And *you* certainly don't have to be blond and breasty to be a potent seductress in your own bedroom.

Your power in the bedroom will come not from your looks, but from the energy that goes into your performance. Every professional stripper learns this lesson.

And the more energy you give out, the more you can expect in return.

"New York, New York"

It was a typical Saturday night in a strip club and the place was packed. The clientele were mainly young men in their early thirties out for a howl. The energy in the room had been elevated by the great performers who had gone on before. It was nearly midnight, and I was starting to feel tired. Reflecting on the two shows I had done earlier that day, I wondered what it would be like to work nine to five in an office again. What was I doing with my life?

"Fifteen minutes to show time, Ciara," the disk jockey told me (referring to me by my stage name), abruptly ending my self-absorbed thoughts. That's the downside of being a headliner, I realized: You have to go on last just when you feel like turning in.

"Gentlemen," I heard the disc jockey announce. "Coming up in just a few minutes, we have the lovely, the talented, the sexy Ms. Nude and Show Girl of the Year, Ms. Ciara Love." The temperature in the room went up another three degrees.

Backstage I was attending to the last details of my costume. I had chosen my "formal suit" of white satin tuxedo jacket and white spandex pants featuring black satin trim from the knees down. My imitation tuxedo shirt and black bow tie were complemented by three-inch black patent-leather stilettos, a pop-up top hat, and a stylish walking cane. Attitude! Attitude! Attitude! I kept thinking to myself.

"Please welcome to the stage, Ms. Ciara Love!" The moment I placed my first foot on the stage, I could feel the electricity from the room surge through my body. The song "Puttin' on the Ritz" was playing, and I felt hot! I did an easy strut across the stage, popped open my hat, and placed it on my head with flair. Using the tip of my cane and a look of disdain, I poked a man sitting too close in the front row. The crowd laughed. This music had attitude built right in, and I knew it well.

By the time I got to my third song, "New York, New York," I was so pumped, I felt like climbing the Empire State Building myself. The crowd's cheering and howling told me they felt it, too. The song ended and I gracefully took a bow. But the crowd couldn't be managed, and weren't about to let the feeling end. They were screaming and clapping and shouting, "More, more, more!" I still had my floor show left to do, but they wanted an encore now. The disk jockey caught the spirit.

"Do you all wanna hear that song again?" he

shouted into the mike. "YEAHHH," came the reply. So I danced to "New York, New York" one more time. When I finished, they did the same thing. They cheered for more. As I stood in front of them with disbelief on my face, one by one, the entire room stood up clapping and cheering me on for another encore. Suddenly, the lump I found in my throat made it hard to swallow. I blinked away the tears that started to trickle down my cheeks. Needless to say, this doesn't happen to exotic dancers often.

I reached for my floor-show blanket and asked the crowd, "Which side of the room wants to see my floor show up real close?" You couldn't hear the music over their roaring. I put my blanket down and the song "Masquerade" began to play. Now the audience became as attentive as they had been boisterous only moments before. The front row had their chins forward nearly to the stage, and all eyes in the room were on me. It was the most touching performance from an audience I have ever seen!

I realize now what inspired the audience that night. They were moved by the character I portrayed and the energy I conveyed while I was on that stage. In a word, ATTITUDE! All they wanted to do was watch me perform. I was hot not because I was naked, but because I was performing for *them*.

—A Rose by Any Other Name . . .—

Professional exotic dancers create stage names for themselves for three reasons:

1. to protect themselves and their families from unwanted attention offstage
2. to enhance or evoke a stage persona
3. to grab our attention and make us smile

Since your career as a seductress/stripper is likely going to remain a domestic affair for the foreseeable future, reasons 1 and 3 won't be a concern. The wild new creature that is beginning to emerge in you needs a name, however, and the one on your driver's license is completely inadequate. You need a stripper name for your new persona.

The best stripper names take a distinguishing characteristic and put it front stage center. These five classics speak for themselves:

Chesty Morgan
Busty Monroe
Annie Ample
Tiffany Towers
Miss 46 Ann How

Luscious Lips Loren was a tall black woman I met on the road who had very distinct facial features, especially her large, luscious lips. With great care she would overpaint them to bring out her natural charm. Other strippers have invented names that draw attention to their thighs, hair, hips, and skin. Do you or your partner have a favorite body part of yours that could serve as the basis for your new name?

Sex and eating share the distinction of being powerful, primal, and sensual pleasures. It comes as no surprise therefore that food, particularly fruit and sweets, figure prominently in any list of stripper names. Anna Banana worked some of the clubs I worked when I began. She would consume bananas onstage in a deep, erotic way. Men found that Cupcake Cassidy filled her cups with double the sweetness.

Other names seek to create an impression of wealth or luxury. Mercedes and Porsche are two from the automotive world I have encountered. Cristal and Chanel borrow from expensive products. Sherri Champagne did an intoxicating act in a giant wineglass complete with bubbles.

If you are still stuck for ideas, I have a formula for you to try. In the left of two columns, list the following: your favorite fruit, a dessert topping, your most coveted luxury item, your best body part, your invisible childhood friend, and your favorite childhood toy. In the right-hand column place the last name of your first boyfriend, an imported wine or alcoholic beverage, and the town in which you were born.

Scan back and forth to see if you have a fit. Look for alliteration (same first letter) or a rhyme. Reverse their relative positions or take two names from one column if that helps.

You should be able to create something with a good rhythmic feel. When I tried this on my friends, they came up with some good ones:

Easy-Bake Shortcake

Gams El Grande

Ms. Chocolate Eclair

Sally Sterling Silver

Most of all, find a name that is fun and comfortable!

Sharing Fantasies

The popular movie *True Lies* has 5 a subplot that perfectly illustrates the value of communication between a couple. The key scene in this subplot involves the wife's first attempt at stripping. Much of this scene is relevant to the subject of this book, so I shall describe it here.

Jamie Lee Curtis is a bored wife with a mundane office job. Her husband, no less than Arnold Schwarzenegger, works in computer sales and is frequently away from home due to business travel. Or so she thinks. In actual fact he is a top international spy working for an undisclosed agency. In typical Schwarzenegger style, he saves the world almost daily. None of this is known to her. Meanwhile, desperate for some excitement in her life, she reads spy books and fantasizes. She soon falls prey to a used-car salesman pretending to be a secret agent of some sort. Our "spy" claims to need her and so involves her in his imaginary plots. She cooperates even when it looks as though things will wind up in the bedroom, not because she wants an affair, but because she craves the excitement. So that's the irony: Her husband doesn't know she wants excitement, and she doesn't know her husband is exciting.

Nevertheless, they almost get a chance to act out their fantasies. Our husband Arnold learns of this affair and uses his best team of spies to thwart it. Without revealing his involvement, Arnold conscripts her support for his side in the spy game. Partly to reward her, but mostly to teach her a lesson, he sends her off on a mission. Curtis must pose as a prostitute in order to plant a bug on a man's hotel telephone. All she knows about the stranger she must meet is that he doesn't want sex, he only wants to watch. Our stranger, of course, will be Arnold.

According to his plans, her reward will come when she finds out it is her husband she has entertained, not a stranger. But an unexpected reward comes his way, too. He sees his wife blossom as a seductress while he watches from the shadows, giving her instructions on what to do to be seductive. Ironically, once again both their fantasies are about to come true, without their knowing, when the real bad guys burst in to put an end to their liaison.

Our spy has learned that his wife, the plain Jane he left at home only this morning, is, deep down, really a hot tamale. She learns that her boring, never-at-home salesman husband is a major spy on the hunt for international terrorists. Because they never shared their innermost feelings in the first place, they almost missed learning that they were exactly what the other fantasized about all along. It would have been much easier for them if they had just been clear about their desires up front. (But then we would have missed out on the best scene in the movie!)

Honest communication should be your primary approach to collecting the information you need to learn your partner's fantasy. Think of the task ahead of you as harmless intelligence gathering. Your mission, should you decide to accept it, will be to design a seduction fantasy that drives you both wild. By reading this book, you are already getting in touch with your own unexpressed desires; now it's time to learn about his. Like you, he may have more than one. With luck you can find a match. When you do, concentrate your efforts there. Above all don't treat it as work, make it fun.

Your husband or boyfriend may not be an international man of mystery, but there may be more to him than you realized. You don't necessarily know his fantasy life until you dig for it. I ask my students if they know exactly what their partners' sexual fantasies are. Most have only a vague notion at best.

If you complain that he never gives you flowers, ask yourself if you have ever told him how much you enjoy flowers. Men don't have ESP, and sometimes they need a little idea planted in their heads. So pick your moment carefully and communicate *your* fantasies to *him*. At the very least he may be more sensitive to your desires the next time you make love. Better than that, it may open a new conversation in which he reveals a bit of his inner life. Revealing your fantasies gives him permission and the safety to share his fantasies with you.

It may not be necessary to discover if he has an elaborate secret scenario all cooked up in his fantasy mind. If it involves someone else, like that cute young doctor he met while having his physical last month, he won't tell you anyway. Like a detective on a case, remember that even little bits of information can be instructive. Often they contain hidden clues. Your second approach will be to look for images, props, or items of clothing that crop up repeatedly in his conversation or actions.

The Clues

Your man probably has favorite female movie stars or TV stars whom he comments on. What sort of roles do they play? What sorts of things do they do, and how do they interact with the male leads? Who are his favorite male leads? Does he fancy himself James Bond or Han Solo? Dr. Evil or Mr. Spock? Does he have a favorite genre of movie, such as Westerns, musical comedy, or film noir? Is there a specific scene he plays over and over on the VCR? When you two are out in public, take note of the kinds of women he is trying not to let you see that he notices. These are the sorts of clues that can give you an insight into the images in his head.

Does he seem more amorous when you go away for that fishing vacation? Maybe it's the feeling of being outdoors that he likes. Or maybe it's the sight and smell of those thigh-high rubber hip waders you wear. Does he still talk about how the two of you made out in the back-seat at the old drive-in or in the washroom of Flight 109? Perhaps the wickedness of doing it where you might get caught appeals to him. Look for clues like this to determine what props or settings may work in your seduction scene.

At the very least you should be able to pick out the clothes he likes to see on women. Chances are good that he has made his feelings known on that already. Does he always compliment you when you wear that long leather coat? Does he own a lot of leather himself? These could be clues to an undisclosed leather fetish, for example. Does he go wild when he sees you in shorts and T-shirt, or do you get the most attention on those formal occasions when you bring out the evening gown and heels?

How does he feel about lingerie? All men have opinions on that. Does he like garters and stockings? Merry widows or matching push-up bra and panties? Does the Sears catalog naturally fall open to the page that shows negligees? Think back to the time before mortgages and dental work for the children seemed so important. Did he ever buy you something that you never wore because you exchanged it for something much more sensible? Now, *that* is a clue.

Your attempt to obtain this information will naturally be much easier if your partner is a creative contributor and knows you are planning a seduction scene. Even in that case, don't tell him all the details. There should always be an element of surprise. You'll both get a bigger kick out of it that way. On the other hand, if you plan to surprise him completely with your seduction scene, then you have the extra burden of choosing just the right time.

Choosing the Time

Make observations about your partner and find out what situations put him in a good mood or a bad mood so that when you are ready to perform, so is he. Is he up after he scores a new deal, or is he exhausted? Is he down around his birthday or during the Christmas holidays, or do these occasions make him more outgoing and friendly? Is he a morning or a night person? Is he preoccupied and disinterested in you during the buildup to the Super Bowl, or is he a boiling cauldron of testosterone that threatens to scald you? Learn his cycles.

Many women assume that men are always up for sex. This simply is not the case. Men's libidos go up and down just like ours, for many of the same

TIP

UNDER NO CIRCUMSTANCES TRY TO GET HIS ATTENTION BY STANDING IN FRONT OF THE TV IN YOUR SEXIEST OUTFIT IN THE HOPE OF SEDUCING HIM. IF YOU DERAIL HIS ATTENTION TO THE BIG GAME, EXPECT A TRAIN WRECK.

reasons—mainly external stresses. In one case I know, this belief in perpetual male horniness caused a woman (not a student of mine) to misjudge her husband's eagerness with unfortunate consequences.

A gentleman I know practices law for a prominent law firm. His practice puts him in regular contact with demanding celebrities and the deals he negotiates can be volatile. One day a couple of deals ran into trouble and other things conspired to make it a day from hell. At home his marriage was in trouble, adding to the stress he felt. After jumping through hoops all day for his clients, he arrived home late, tired and hungry. When he walked in the door, his wife was waiting in her sexiest lingerie and nightgown, romantic music was playing, and the table was set for a candlelight dinner for two. She was ready to seduce him. But he was in no mood to be seduced.

Contrary to the popular myth, his only thought was, Oh no! Now I have to put on a performance for her, too. He simply was not in the mood and was too tired to keep his feelings from showing. He still loved her and understood the effort she had made, but more than anything needed the night off—completely off. Regrettably, her good intentions could not overcome the bad timing.

With a little homework she may have discovered

that this was not the best night to plan a romantic evening. A simple thing like a phone call can prevent the disappointment that comes when things don't go your way. You've heard it before: All good things are worth waiting for, and timing is everything.

I believe my friend's wife made another mistake when she sought to use seduction instead of communication to revive a failing relationship. Seduction and stripping for your partner are best for healthy, happy couples who are both on the same page. The only way to get on the same page is to communicate your thoughts and hopes with each other. Don't use the techniques explained in this book to fix a broken relationship. Use them to enhance an already good one.

A woman I heard about through a dancer friend learned this lesson the hard way, despite a seduction idea that would have been foolproof in better circumstances. Her idea started in the kitchen. Taking the notion of peeling literally, she decided to use Saran Wrap for her costume. She started at her feet and wrapped and wrapped until she ran out at her neck.

When her husband got home, he was surprised all right. She turned on some music and began peeling layer and layer of plastic wrap off until there was nothing left but her. This is one case where she would have been better off using a non–name brand, though. Because the good food wrap sticks so well, she found it difficult knowing where one piece ended and another began.

That difficulty may have slowed her show down a bit, but it wasn't what eventually killed the marriage. She didn't get the big reaction she was expecting for her performance, and that left her feeling uneasy. She had made the same mistake of trying to spice up a failing relationship. It was understandable, though—her husband had recently confessed to having a brief affair. Sometimes people take drastic measures and do things they would not normally do when they feel their partner is slipping away. Don't wait too long. We can only wonder what the outcome might have been had this woman tried her seduction scene before her husband had his affair.

The Doctor/Patient Relationship

There are far more good stories out there, stories that show how a little surprise, properly timed, can keep a good relationship fresh. One woman I know was able to use her detailed knowledge of her boyfriend's personality to set a seduction trap. Matthew and Nancy have a relationship that has been going strong since they started dating three years ago. They talk openly and often about their needs and wants.

Nancy has a few health problems. Fortunately, Matthew is very attentive and comforting when she isn't feeling well, almost to the point of behaving like a doctor. Nancy knew from past experience that whenever she was sick, Matthew dropped everything to be there for her.

Nancy's only complaint was that Matthew worked too hard and they couldn't spend enough time alone together. Knowing this, Matthew surprised Nancy one day with a trip for two to Florida. She didn't believe they were actually taking this vacation together until she boarded the plane.

After arriving at their hotel around noon, the couple unpacked and headed straight for the ocean to swim and laze on the beach for the remainder of the afternoon. They finished the day with a romantic dinner. The evening was to be a quiet one in their room with a movie. Nancy went into the bedroom while Matthew prepared the popcorn and set up the movie.

When Nancy didn't come out of the bedroom, Matthew got worried and called in to her, "Hey, Nancy, what's taking you so long?" She moaned and said she wasn't feeling very well. He came into the bedroom to see her lying in bed bundled up under the covers showing only her long, sad face. She told him she was sick, and perhaps she had gotten too much sun on the first day out.

Matthew started playing the doctor, exactly as Nancy knew he would. First he got a cold cloth for her head. In a weak and whiny voice she apologized, "I'm sorry, Doctor, for spoiling our first vacation together." Thinking his vacation was ruined, Matthew began to feel sick, too. With deepening concern, he left the room to get her something to drink. When he returned with a glass of juice, instead of drinking it she flung back the covers.

There she was, dressed in a hospital gown and stilettos, with garters and the tops of her stockings showing below her raised hem. Springing from the bed, she pushed the play button on the tape player and started a seductive strip to the song "Doctor, Doctor." Matthew had been fooled but he was a happy guy. This was her way of paying him back for all his "medical" attention. She surprised him and he loved it!

Now and then I encounter a woman who objects to my approach. "Why should I be the one to do all the work and plan a seduction?" goes the reasoning. It's a familiar complaint: Why do women have to take responsibility for the relationship?

Well, what is wrong with being proactive? You have two choices. You can do nothing and let your romantic life slip into senility, or you can take some responsibility and take action. If you want the results, you need to take the risks. Of course, romance should be give-and-take. So start by giving a little. Once you start the ball rolling, I'm betting your partner will catch the hint and start surprising you with a bit of giving of his own.

Bookstores have shelves of books in the self-help section proclaiming the value of good communication in a relationship. No doubt you will start to see some of the benefits they promise in your relationship as a result of your efforts. But your immediate goal should be to identify what turns you on and look for a match in your partner's fantasy life. Everything you do from here on in to plan your seduction scene will be informed by the knowledge you gain. In the chapters that follow you will choose a role and a costume, plan the music and set the stage, and most important, learn some very sexy moves.

Like our couple in *True Lies*, you and your partner may have perfectly compatible romantic desires without knowing it. Here is your chance to make your fantasies come true.

Choosing a Role

One October, many years ago, I **6** stood with my friend Rosie in an aisle of the local department store. We were eight years old. Before us, on hangers, was an array of plastic Halloween costumes, such as a witch, vampire, princess, ghost, etc. Accessories sat on shelves nearby.

"Who do you want to be?"

"I want to be a princess, because princesses are pretty and everyone loves them," my friend explained.

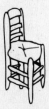 "But you were a princess last year," I pointed out.

The princess-to-be

explained how she had kept the dress her mother made from a fancy old nightgown. I recalled the lace fringe at the sleeves and hem. She described how the tiara on display before us would look great with the earrings she had made from her grandma's old jewelry.

"I'm gonna be the best princess ever this year."

Rosie wasn't in the habit of asking what I was going to be, so I offered, softly but firmly, "For this Halloween, I'm gonna be a secret agent like James Bond."

"You?" My friend registered her disbelief.

Our mothers appeared at this moment to claim us. Rosie got her tiara, and I got the secret wristwatch I had my eye on—the one with the flip-up top that became a communicator. For the next few weeks Rosie and I worked on our costumes. She worked with her mother sewing beads and fastening stones to her costume; I worked with my brother to make pretend radios with wire coat hangers for antennas, along with other gadgets and secret weapons.

On Halloween night the princess looked adorable in her elaborate dress and jewelry, with her hair pulled up under the tiara. We had even applied some makeup to her face. I looked pretty ordinary by comparison. I was wearing dark pants and a shirt with a tie. My main preoccupation was the jacket I borrowed from my brother. I needed lots of inside pockets and places to hide my gadgets. Wraparound sunglasses were the only external clue indicating that I was an international agent, not merely a child in her brother's clothes.

I didn't envy my friend Rosie and her costume for long once we started on our rounds of candy collection. My costume didn't restrict my movements, and I was free to act like a daring and confident spy. I took charge, helping Rosie up and down the steps, an act made difficult by her long hemline and slippers with heels. Acting the lady, my friend let me reach for the candy and distribute it between the two bags. What a ball we had changing our characters!

Right now, you are faced with decisions much like a little girl looking at costumes in a department store. Who am I going to be? What shall I wear? You have a big event coming up and you are excited. Like the two girls described above, you understand that all this will take some advanced planning. Also like the two girls, you know that your efforts will be rewarded. The only difference is, now that we're grown up, we go for bigger and better treats!

There are a number of important lessons to be learned from this Halloween story as we prepare for our night of seduction.

1. *The roles we pick determine the costumes we wear or, vice versa, the costumes we pick determine the roles we play.*

2. *These roles come in two broad categories: dominant and submissive.*

3. *Playacting is fun, no matter who you decide to be.*

4. *Not everything you need is available at the local store. Costumes can be put together combining store-bought items with things you already have at home, stitched together with a lot of creativity.*

Before you start planning your performance, think about the role you will be playing, or in the words of a child, "Who do you want to be?" Use your own fantasies as a guide. They will help you get into your role. Be creative. Be entertaining. Remember that you don't have to get naked and sleazy to do this. For all of you natural-born actors, this is your chance to play your biggest part yet. Fun and playfulness are key ingredients.

When I ask the students in my workshops for roles a woman might play in her seduction scene, the response is enthusiastic. As my students call out their suggestions, I drop them into the two categories, dominant and submissive. As it turns out, these are the same two categories exotic dancers have been using to shape their acts since stripping began.

DOMINANT	SUBMISSIVE
Catwoman	Schoolgirl
Cop	French Maid
Tiger	Domestic Cat
Zena, the Warrior Princess	Geisha Girl
Dominatrix	Hooker
Bitch Boss	Slave/Harem Girl
Devil	Angel
Nurse	Nurse
Secretary	Secretary

Note how the roles of nurse and secretary can be placed in both categories. I guess it just depends on who is giving the orders where you work! The nurse and secretary costumes, and perhaps the tiger/cat costume, can do double service. The music and attitude you bring to your performance will determine whether you're the boss or just the help.

If you are the one who dominates in your relationship outside the bedroom, you may want to choose a softer role for this occasion and allow your partner to have the upper hand. This may be the opportunity he has been waiting for to express himself more freely. Or, if he generally calls the shots, he may welcome a take-charge dominatrix in the bedroom. Your communication and research should help you make this decision. The dominance and submission that goes on in a relationship is a subtle and shifting thing. Be honest with yourself. I won't believe you if you tell me he is always the boss. In the bedroom as elsewhere, it pays to understand how the dynamic between the two of you works. Many couples try on different roles, taking turns being dominant and submissive. Sometimes they decide one way works best for both of them; sometimes they keep alternating.

I also create a third list for my class. A number of roles are neutral on the dominance scale. For example:

NEUTRAL

Belly Dancer

Mrs. Santa Claus

Clown

Cowgirl/boy

You Can Leave Your Hat On

When wearing these "neutral" outfits, you don't have a built-in dominance or submissiveness to guide your approach. So remember, however you play it, you must always be seductive. Neutral roles do lend themselves especially well to enhancement by props. With a little imagination, this list of neutral roles can be expanded endlessly, as the following description of show ideas demonstrates. Any person who wears a uniform can assume a role. You may decide, once you really embrace it, that your role has more potential if you push it into either the dominant or submissive camps. Just think of how you might deliver those UPS parcels now!

Keep in mind that it isn't always what your partner sees that gets him going; sometimes it's what he can't see. A lot can be done with just the simple things on hand, a little imagination, and a lot of attitude, as a scene in the movie *9 ½ Weeks* demonstrates.

In the scene I'm thinking of, Kim Basinger does a striptease for Mickey Rourke, who watches from the couch while he nibbles on popcorn. The glass doors to the apartment balcony have been opened to give the appearence of a stage. Kim starts her act on the balcony but out of sight beyond the entranceway.

The music playing is Joe Cocker's "You Can Leave Your Hat On." Handcuffs and a riding crop are the first things Mickey's character sees projecting from offstage, giving him a taste of what is to come. Kim's arms and legs appear seductively one by one. Eventually she is there in the entranceway but coyly hiding behind the louvered blinds, which she uses to alternately reveal and conceal herself. Her costume is a fedora and a belted trench coat that she plays with erotically, allowing us to guess that she is wearing little or nothing underneath. Above all else, her attitude sells the performance. The show is clearly all about playfulness and fun. The looks on Mickey's face register amusement, lust, and approval. I recommend you watch this film for inspiration.

Some Show Ideas

I've polled my dancer friends and searched through my own memories to compile this list of show ideas. A list of song titles accompanies each description. This is simply a list of possibilities. If you don't see something you can use, these ideas should at least jump-start your imagination.

FIRE SHOW

I have seen many dancers attempt fire shows. One dancer came onstage in an actual fireman's jacket for her first song. She did a fire-eating routine during her third song and rubbed a burning torch all over her body for her finale. Note: Do not attempt this in your home unless you have the proper training! Somehow I suspect this is further than most of you want to go, but if the "fire" theme interests you, know that it can be done without the real thing. I came up with a "Hellfire" theme in which I dressed as a devil with little horns, a red tail, and a pitchfork. I used the appropriate music, but no real flames.

1. Fire	*Arthur Brown*
2. Go to Hell	*Alice Cooper*
3. Evil Ways	*Santana*
4. Black Magic Woman	*Santana*

CLOWN SHOW

When I did this show, two bouncers carried me onstage tucked inside a large wooden box that was full of helium-filled balloons. As the audience waited for me to make my entrance from offstage, I released a balloon from inside the box every time Judy Collins sang the line, "Where are the clowns?" Toward the end of the first song I slowly emerged from the box holding the last balloon to the lyric "Making my entrance again, with my usual flair." My clown outfit consisted of large bloomer pants and a baggy matching top in blue and white checks. The collar was designed to stay around my neck when the rest of the outfit came off.

During my second song, "The Tears of a Clown," I danced around with a hankie drying my tears. When

Smokey sang, "When there's no one around," I would pull out the waistband of my baggy pants and peek inside like a lonely little clown. Then I used a cane to gently poke some unsuspecting member of the front row in his crotch. I continued to entertain with simple magic tricks. The audience watched like entranced six-year-olds.

1. *Send In the Clowns*	*Judy Collins*
2. *The Tears of a Clown*	*Smokey Robinson*
3. *Everybody Loves a Clown*	*Gary Lewis and the Playboys*
4. *See the Funny Little Clown*	*Bobby Goldsboro*
5. *Goodbye Cruel World*	*James Darren*
6. *Don't Cry Out Loud*	*Melissa Manchester*

GANGSTER SHOW

In this number I blasted onto stage dressed in a black trench coat and fedora. The machine gun in my hands was a squirt gun filled with a harmless, water-soluble blue dye. The businessmen freaked out when they saw the blue water hitting their white shirts. Thinking the stains were permanent, they wondered how they would hide the evidence. How could they explain this one when they got home?

1. *The Friends of Mr. Cairo*   *Jon & Vangelis*

2. *Dirty Deeds Done*   *AC/DC*
   Dirt Cheap

3. *Another One Bites the Dust*   *Queen*

4. *Peter Gunn*   *Henry Mancini, Blues*
   Brothers

LITTLE-GIRL SHOW

Boy, was I cute: pigtails tied with colorful bows, and rosy cheeks and freckles. I wore layers and layers of crinoline under a pretty floral-printed skirt with ruffles around the bottom. Underneath were bloomers, and above, a frilly white blouse. Little white gloves on my hands held a large lollipop on which my tongue demonstrated its talents. A giant pacifier around my neck was a substitute when the lollipops were unavailable.

By the time I stripped down to my crinoline, I moved close to the front row and lifted it over some guy's head. I then reached under it and pulled a sucker from my panties. Under the crinoline and out of the audience's view, I unwrapped the sucker and stuck it in the fellow's mouth. When I let him up for air, the audience assumed he had helped himself to the candy. Bad boy.

1. *Candy Girl*	*New Edition*
2. *My Boy Lollipop*	*Millie Small*
3. *Candy Man*	*Sammy Davis Jr.*
4. *Brand New Key*	*Melanie*
5. *Playground in My Mind*	*Clint Holmes*
6. *Go Away Little Girl*	*Steve Lawrence, Donny Osmond*
7. *Come Back When You Grow Up*	*Bobby Vee*

JAILBIRD SHOW

Here my costume featured a striped black-and-white miniskirt with matching striped jacket. A little pillbox hat sat on my head, held in place by an elastic band behind my ears and under my hair. My ankle pulled a plastic ball and chain and my wrists wore handcuffs. The fun started when I got someone to break me loose from the handcuffs.

1. *Bad*	*Michael Jackson*
2. *Chain Gang*	*Sam Cooke*
3. *Naughty, Naughty*	*John Parr*
4. *Jailhouse Rock*	*Elvis Presley*

TIP

RAGS TO RICHES

The local discount store had everything I needed for the "rags" part of my costume at only seven dollars. I took a baggy suit, tore it in spots, and painted it to look dirty. An old shirt and tie and black gloves with the fingers cut out completed the look. For the "riches" part of the routine, I shed the hobo threads to reveal a beautiful black sequin bra and panties.

1. *Mr. Bojangles* — *Jerry Jeff Walker*
2. *King of the Road* — *Roger Miller*
3. *Poor Side of Town* — *Johnny Rivers*
4. *Money Changes Everything* — *Cyndi Lauper*
5. *Money* — *Pink Floyd*
6. *Loan Me a Dime* — *Boz Scaggs*

SECRETARY SHOW

A simple but well-fitted black-and-white pinstripe skirt and jacket cover a naughty secret self that likes push-up bras, garters, and stockings in this scenario. During "9 to 5," I strode around onstage drinking coffee out of a mug, looking lazy and bored. For the second song, I passed around little notepads with sexual questions written on them. One of notes I gave to the lunch crowd asked, "How big is yours?" The men never hesitated to respond with funny answers. One guy drew a penis on the front of the notepaper that continued around to the other side with the note "There's not enough room."

1. 9 to 5	Dolly Parton
2. She Works Hard for the Money	Donna Summer
3. Take This Job and Shove It	Johnny Paycheck
4. Out of Work	Gary U.S. Bonds
5. Dreams of the Everyday Housewife	Glen Campbell
6. You Are My Lady	Freddie Jackson

CHRISTMAS SHOW

My all-time favorite show! The regulars looked forward every year to their turn to retrieve the little candy canes I gave away. I wore a pair of red tights with a red jacket that I made out of an old red bathrobe. I trimmed all the edges in white fur and made a little red hat with the leftover fabric and the same white fur. I wore a thick black belt *à la* Santa Claus, and red-beaded bra and panties underneath on which I hung my candy canes. After I took my bra off, I hung candy canes from my nipples. Naughty or nice, every willing volunteer had to work for his gift.

1. *Feliz Navidad*	*Jose Feliciano*
2. *Jingle Bell Rock*	*Bobby Helms*
3. *White Christmas*	*Bing Crosby, et al.*
4. *Christmas Time*	*Bryan Adams*
5. *Santa Claus Is Back in Town*	*Elvis Presley*

CAT SHOW

For this endeavour I had someone paint my face to look like the little cat faces that children get when they go to fairs. My bra, G-string, armbands, and leggings were made from soft, fun fur. The center of attraction to this outfit was the long furry tail I wore. I held it as I pranced around the stage, pausing on occasion to lick it lovingly. Making my way over to a customer, I asked,

"Do you want a piece of tail?" He would gulp and say, "Yeah," with enthusiasm. Then, from a slit in the tail, I would pull out a piece of fluff about an inch in diameter that was sprayed with my perfume and hand it over to the surprised guy.

Ten years after the club in which I invented this show closed, I bumped into one of the regulars. He recognized me right away and pulled out his wallet and showed me a piece of tail that he had saved as a souvenir. It smelled more like his wallet than my perfume by then, but the thought was touching all the same.

1. *What's New Pussycat?*	*Tom Jones*
2. *Stray Cat Strut*	*Stray Cats*
3. *Year of the Cat*	*Al Stewart*

COWGIRL

What can I say? Get a cowboy hat and a pair of cowboy boots, cut the rear out of a pair of old blue jeans, or buy yourself a pair of tear-away fringed pants with a matching vest, and off you go. I have seen dancers wear just about anything for this show, but you can't do it without the hat. That is a must!

1. *Rodeo Song*	*Showdown*
2. *Wasn't That a Party?*	*The Rovers*
3. *Thirsty Ears*	*Powder Blues Band*
4. *Are There Any More Real Cowboys?*	*Neil Young*

OLD-LADY SHOW

A friend of mine started her show dressed up as an old lady. She tied a white wig onto her head with a handkerchief and wore thick black-rimmed glasses to conceal her eyes. Her dress was a light blue flowered print with a zipper down the front (the kind that looked like an apron). Her black purse hung around her elbow and her hose stopped just above her calves. She walked onstage carrying a shopping bag, of course, and a boom box that played the song "Wild Thing." She played with herself and felt herself up as she attempted to dance to the music. When the clothes, wig, etc., came off, she revealed the blond, blue-eyed former Ms. Nude Sweden she really was—much to the relief of the audience.

1. *Wild Thing*	*The Troggs*
2. *The Little Old Lady from Pasadena*	*Jan and Dean*

3. Second Hand Rose	*Barbra Streisand*
4. Young Girl	*Gary Puckett and the Union Gap*

RAIN SET

I started my rain set covered by a pink plastic see-through raincoat and umbrella. Tricks with the umbrella provided the interest during the first song. I remained hidden behind the umbrella for most of the floor show, tossing the G-string into the crowd as the final gesture.

1. Singing in the Rain	*Gene Kelly*
2. Raindrops Keep Falling on My Head	*B. J. Thomas*
3. Raindrops	*Dee Clark*
4. Lightnin' Strikes	*Lou Christie*

Above all, these shows demonstrate playfulness and a sense of fun—two things welcome in everyone's romantic life. There are more than enough ideas to revive in you the Halloween spirit you felt as a young girl. Take a chance and enjoy yourself!

What to Wear, What to Wear . . .

Go to your room and open your *7*

underwear drawer. Is cotton the sole fabric

you find? Does everything match now that

it's all off-white to light gray in color? Is

the only metal in any of your bras a safety

pin? Do you have no idea what size you

are because all the tags have long since

disappeared or faded into oblivion? Can

you even remember which parts of your

underwear once used to stretch? Do you

have a piece that you never wear because,

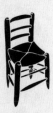 frankly, you can't figure out

what part of your body it's

supposed to cover? Do you

think they call it support hose because it's designed to hold *you* up? Is there anything in your drawer you haven't worn since you pretended to be delighted that your partner bought it for you? Are you proud of the fact that you save money by wearing two pairs of panty hose at the same time, each with only one leg remaining? If you've answered yes to any of these questions, then it's time for a lingerie makeover.

All men love lingerie. They would wear it themselves if they could. Some even do. Some men go nuts for garters and stockings. Some like skimpy bra and panty sets, while others prefer teddies. A solid contingent feels that merry widows, corsets, and bustiers are the greatest inventions to come down to us from the past. Still others like the sensuality of transparent nightgowns, peignoirs, or baby-doll pajamas. If you have done your research as outlined in Chapter 5 (or if you've known him long enough to have been told over and over), you probably have a good idea what turns his crank.

Armed with this information, and with a good idea of the role you will be playing, it's time to go shopping. For starters, it may not be necessary to leave your house. Several catalogs exist specializing in lingerie. Frederick's of Hollywood and Victoria's Secret are the two best known, but there are many others. Some will have pages actually devoted to fantasy costumes. The catalog from a local importer on my desk at the moment shows a "Police Woman" set (with baton and handcuffs!), a "Cheerleader" set, a "Schoolgirl" set, a "Scottish Dancer" set, a "Pussy Cat" set (my favorite; I like the tail), and a "Prisoner of Love" set, for example. The rest of the pages show everything I have ever thought of, and a few things I haven't. Get on the Internet, and get on some mailing lists.

I live in a major urban center. Every fall the "Everything to Do With Sex" show comes to the convention hall downtown. In one stop I can collect dozens of catalogs and inspect the merchandise up close. This is a wonderful opportunity to see what's available. Chances are there is some sort of specialty store in your hometown you didn't know about. They can tell you if a similar show is coming to the urban center nearest you.

Suggest to your partner that he come along. It should be a good way to do some research on his preferences as well as your own. If he has already made plans to go to the auto-parts store for a new ballast resistor, then ask a girlfriend. These shows are more fun to attend in pairs or groups.

While some women prefer the anonymity of ordering over the phone or on the Internet, others appreciate the help and personal attention they get when they shop in person. Some reputable upscale lingerie stores actually have professional bra fitters who will come right into the fitting room with you. These women have experience fitting any size and shape of breasts to ensure a comfortable fit and sexy look. You may find their assistance indispensable on your first trip.

In the last ten years I have noticed a lot of specialty stores springing up in my city. Some specialize only in leather (and I don't mean purses and handbags), and many include "adult sex toys" along with their lingerie. I have been in a few that deal only in high-heeled shoes and boots. One of the more established specialty leather stores in my city features their own designer fetish wear, and holds an annual fashion show. The media covers the event and attendance rises every year. So do their sales. I like to think this success is because couples are communicating better and having more fun with each other. If you're in one of these specialty stores in your town, find out if they participate in any fashion shows.

My point is this: It's getting easier and easier to find just what you are looking for no matter where you live. You will likely have lots of company when you go looking, and there is no need to feel embarrassed. (Wait until you surprise your boss in one of these stores—I did.) The only risk you face is going to be short supply. So start your search now.

TIP

DRAG QUEENS NEVER TAKE BEING A WOMAN FOR GRANTED. CONSULT A LOCAL DRAG QUEEN FOR ADVICE. WHEN IT COMES TO DRESSING FOR EFFECT, SHE'S DONE IT ALL, HONEY!

Do-It-Yourself Outfits

All of this is well and good, you say, but "I don't have the money to do this kind of shopping. After all, I'm only going to wear this outfit on the weekends when the kids are at their grandparents'." I understand, I understand.

During my twenty years as an exotic dancer I sometimes had to come up with as many as five different costumes a day, and change them regularly as I added new routines. This could get very expensive if I shopped in specialty stores for everything. Like all feature dancers, I learned how to be frugal when it came to costumes. Even Gypsy Rose Lee used to make her own costumes from old curtains. And so second-hand clothing stores will be your home away from home. You will develop a whole new attitude toward old-fashioned girdles.

A thorough tour through my closet reveals a treasure trove of goodies acquired over the years from secondhand stores and consignment shops. The most expensive piece cost maybe thirty-five dollars or so; most were under twenty dollars. All of them could be worked into a costume with a little imagination:

Suede: pants, vest, skirt

Leather: pants, skirt, jackets (in several colors)

Footwear: pumps, mules, sandals, and boots with three-inch-plus heels

Nightgown and lace housecoat

Merry widow, bustier

Lace teddy, bras

Clingy dresses in velvet, spandex

Faux fur jacket, stole

Ballet tutu, crinoline

Cowgirl dress and boots

See-through plastic raincoat and umbrella

Sequined tank top

Jewelry: bracelets, snake armband, huge dangly earrings, choker

Accessories: heart-shaped sunglasses, cincher belts, funky hats and purses

Wigs in several styles and colors, including purple

In addition to saving money, you should be able to justify your purchases for practical reasons. Some of the pieces from your costumes could be incorporated into an outfit you wear to go out for dinner or dancing, for example. Or maybe you will want to feel a bit wicked and wear something from your collection under that plain black suit they've seen you in so many times at work.

A good costume is more than the sum of its parts. No matter how successful your shopping has been, there is still more you can do to make your prize pieces stand out from mere clothing. And none of it needs to cost a lot of money. Some sewing skills may be required for these projects. (Wait until you see how useful a glue gun can be for certain costumes!) Enroll your girlfriends to help you with your project if you can. Maybe they have projects of their own they can bring along. It beats playing bridge on Wednesday nights, or making curtains for the spare room no one ever stays in.

Bustiers

Outdated bustiers are a fabulous place to start. You've probably found one in your size at the local secondhand shop for five dollars or so. Now, we all lose an earring from time to time. I know what I do with my leftovers: I shove them in my junk jewelry drawer along with all the other orphan earrings, knotted necklaces, and lonely rhinestones. Go to your own graveyard of gems and pull out those beaded necklaces you were saving until they come back in style (if you are still alive by that time). Choose one whose color will work well with your planned outfit. Pull the beads off the strand and sew them randomly all over the body of the bustier.

If you have a matching pair of earrings that go with the beads, you can glue them on each cup over your nipples. Be sure to use glue and remove any pins or posts from the earrings; you don't want anything sharp *there*. If you only have a single earring, glue it in the center of the bustier, right between the cups as high as it will go. Finish your bustier off with lace around the top, starting from the armpits and wrapping around to where your cleavage looks best.

Bustiers this nice beg to be worn underneath an open jacket or blouse, with pants or a skirt. When you're not wearing it in the bedroom, take it out for dinner or to a cocktail party. Watch the conversation start—or stop—when you enter.

Leather Outfits

TOOLS AND SUPPLIES

One pair of used suede or leather pants

Bra

Stud gun

Metal eyelets

Assorted sizes of metal studs

Scissors

Glue gun

Velcro

Here's a sexy outfit that's easy to make. You'll be glad you picked up those leather or suede pants second-hand for only thirty dollars, even though the legs were two inches too short. Long pants are the hardest garment to strip off gracefully, even for professional dancers, so we're going to make shorts.

Get out your scissors and chop off the legs as short as you dare. Cut a strip off the separated leg piece to use as a choker, two pieces from the ankles to use as arm bands, and two more pieces for ankle bands. The beauty of leather is that you don't have to sew it. Simply fold the leather over and glue it using a hot glue gun or fabric glue. Attach Velcro in the appropriate places to serve as fasteners. Another option is to cut long strips to make laces that will tie the pieces together. Insert eyelets if you plan to have any pieces lace up together. Sewing studs around the pockets adds a nice touch to the front of the shorts. Feel free to add studs to the armbands, ankle bands, and choker, wherever space permits.

That great bra you bought for only five dollars because it goes with the pants will be the top for your new outfit. Cut diamond or heart-shaped motifs from the remaining leather pieces and use your glue gun to fasten them to the front of the bra. No sewing required. Apply studs to match the armbands, ankle bands, and choker, pulling the whole thing together as an outfit. Say, Baby, you're lookin' tough but sweet, and impossible to beat!

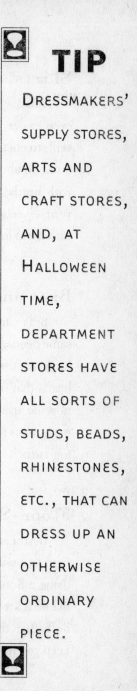

TIP

DRESSMAKERS' SUPPLY STORES, ARTS AND CRAFT STORES, AND, AT HALLOWEEN TIME, DEPARTMENT STORES HAVE ALL SORTS OF STUDS, BEADS, RHINESTONES, ETC., THAT CAN DRESS UP AN OTHERWISE ORDINARY PIECE.

Skirts

You may wish to use a skirt for your outfit. They are even easier to slip out of than shorts. Use your new skills to customize a leather or suede skirt in the manner outlined above. Remember, any skirt can be decorated with beads, rhinestones, or lace. Time to go through your closets, pull out all your outdated clothes, and turn them into seductive treasures.

Bras and Panties

Bras can be made to match a skirt by adding the same beads, rhinestones, or lace. A row of fringe can be hung across the bottom of the cups. The strings of beads that used to hang in doorways in the sixties can now be used to decorate your underwear. There are many ways to match your bra to your panties for a pleasing surprise when your skirt comes off.

Floor-Show Carpet

If you are considering any movements on the floor (and you will be—see Chapter 9), you should consider using a floor-show blanket just like the pros do. These blankets are a lot softer and warmer on the nearly naked body than the hard surface you may be moving on, and keep you from bruising or scraping your knees or other parts. I like to use faux fur. Any fabric store will carry faux fur in a variety of colors. Expect to pay twenty dollars and up depending on size. My favorites are the animal-print or fake mink patterns. You may want to snuggle in it or use it in your performance in some other way. Once again, coordinating your blanket with your costume adds a professional touch. After your performance, you can always put the blanket on your couch and snuggle under it when you watch TV. Your friends will compliment you on it, especially if it also matches your decor.

If you think back to Halloween when you were a child, you can remember how it took weeks to prepare for the big day. Retailers put their costumes and candy on display a month ahead of time. Most of us studied it all wide-eyed, trying to decide what we were going to be. We enrolled our best friends to help us with our costumes and fought with our siblings when they copied our ideas. When adults asked us how we were going to dress, we would holler our answer—"Dracula!"—in a loud and scary voice. Our imaginations would soar and the excitement was more than we could bear. Finally, Halloween night came, and we returned from our rounds with our reward.

Inevitably, the lure of a reward explains why we go

to great lengths for so many things. The reward differs with every effort, and you learn to wait much longer for much more subtle and profound rewards when you become an adult. When we were kids and dressed for Halloween, we went through all that trouble for the candy and goodies that we got at the end of the day. When we dress to enact a sensual performance for our partners, we do it for the endless rewards that come to us long after our seductive evening is over. The trick is to get the treat!

Pasties

No discussion of stripping would be complete without a brief description of pasties. I imagine the pastie was created to get around a technical prohibition on complete nudity. At that time in the affected jurisdictions, G-strings would have to remain in place, too.

I started dancing in the seventies and so just missed the pastie era. All I have to say is OUCH! Regulations governing exotic dancing have always varied from state to state. Thank God pasties weren't required where I first worked. But I did learn to feel—literally—for the dancers who had to deal with this barbaric practice.

My introduction to pasties came in beautiful Hammond, Indiana. I was a feature dancer there and so was entitled to my own private change room. It turned out to be a bathroom just off the kitchen. My dressing mirror was propped up against the large chest freezer.

Knowing I was from out of town, the manager read me the local rules as I prepared for my first show. Then he handed me a strip of stickers that looked like the rolls children have with their favorite characters on them. The flat, round stickers came in two sizes and two colors—small and large and silver or gold. I chose some in each color. I cut a little slit halfway through and turned them into small cones that I stuck on my nipples. Very simple. At the end of the night I peeled them off—along with a layer of skin. The second night

I repeated the same procedure, and by the third day, there was no way I was going to do that again. My nipples were raw!

I happened to be chatting with one of the other girls in their change room and mentioned my pain.

"Oh, didn't you use any cream?"

"Cream?" I asked. "What on earth are you talking about?"

She explained to me that I was supposed to put a little cream on my nipple and allow the sticker to stick only at its edges.

Thanks a lot, I thought. Now you tell me.

That was the downside of having my own change room. I didn't get to share information with the other girls. So I am sharing it with you now. If you plan to go the traditional route and use pasties, make sure you use lots of cream and minimize the adhesion area.

The original pasties came in many different textures, colors, and styles. They matched the elaborate costumes of the feature performers and were held on with a rubbery glue similar to that used to fasten false eyelashes. And, as I learned, strippers did not glue them directly onto the nipple. Some pasties had hanging tassels that matched the dancer's costume. Considerable effort went into the moving of those tassels. A skilled operator could make them move like trained fleas in a jar.

Setting the Stage

In my seventeen-year-old mind, the back row at the drive-in in my boyfriend's father's Impala was the ideal spot for a romantic encounter. Think about all the advantages it has to offer:

1. Privacy: Parents are at home with no transportation. No one wanders past your car to the concession stand when you're in the back row. Other back-row people are much too busy to be looking in your direction.

2. *Wide-screen entertainment: All the latest movies made just for people like you, namely horizontal. Rock and roll between double features. And you've got your own volume control.*

3. *Climate control: Too cold—turn on the engine, turn on the heater. Too hot—open the window. Too smoky—open the vents and turn on the fan.*

4. *Scent: Vinyl upholstery and auto freshener. Yum.*

5. *Smoking permitted: Four—count 'em, four—ashtrays.*

6. *Food: Your choice—with or without butter; Coke and Pepsi.*

7. *Lighting: The dome light covered in pink or blue plastic. Ooooh, sexy.*

8. *Lounge: The front bench seat. Ideal for foreplay.*

9. *Bedroom: The back bench seat. For the follow-through.*

10. *Suspension: The entire passion pad is mounted on springs and rubber!*

Regrettably, those innocent days of simple romantic fulfillment are gone. Your expectations for a romantic evening are greater now. At the very least you would like to be able to stand up without going outside, something not possible at the drive-in. Nevertheless, as you set the stage for your seductive dance and the evening of passion that will follow, many of the same issues that were dealt with so handily by the Impala in the back row are bound to arise.

Privacy

You no longer have to worry about your parents or creepy little brother walking in on you, but the issue of privacy hasn't gone away. You will have to do more than dim the lights and pull the blinds to discourage the neighbors from dropping in to watch the final episode of *Temptation Island*. If you have children at home, make the usual plans. I'm sure you have experience arranging for time off from the kids. Plan for the whole night, even if your seduction is scheduled for the evening only. Send the kids to visit their grandparents, or encourage that sleepover at a friend's they have been talking about. Knowing your kids won't walk in on you will give you the psychological space to relax fully.

If you share an apartment with a roommate, you've probably shared your plans with him or her already. The obvious solution is to trade evenings: You can offer to vacate the premises in the future for his or her big evening with a lover.

Disconnect or otherwise silence all telephones, fax machines, beepers, pagers, and e-mail connections. If necessary, leave one phone activated in a different part of the house and instruct the baby-sitters and any other essential parties to use it *only* in emergencies. The point here is that you want no interruptions or distractions. Just the decision to ignore a ringing phone could be distracting itself. Feed the cat and put the dog in the backyard. Pets have an annoying habit of demanding your attention or getting underfoot at the wrong times.

Lighting

Candlelight is everyone's first choice in seductive lighting. If the light in your seduction room is on a dimmer switch, then you have another option for soft lighting. Sometimes those little night-lights can set the mood if you've got enough of them (and they're not Simpsons characters). If you don't have any night-lights or candles, take a tip from the couple in the Impala we met at the start of this chapter and cover the existing light fixtures with your favorite sheer fabric to soften the light. Choose a color that fits in with the theme for the evening.

Try to resist the temptation to turn the lights down very low or completely off. You need to see what you are doing and whom you are doing it with. Remember, too, how visual men are as erotic creatures. If he's the kind of guy who has installed a draftsman's lamp on the kitchen table so he can get a better look at his steak and onions, then chances are he is going to want the lights a little brighter than you do.

Music

The music you choose is an essential part of the environment you will be creating. The tunes must fit the role you will be playing, and coordinate with any special props you place in the room. Don't choose a piece of music just because you like it. This may seem like the perfect opportunity to dance to your favorite wedding reception tune, like "Copacabana," but if your costume includes leather and whips, maybe you should give Barry Manilow a pass. Likewise, you wouldn't decorate the room with your favorite stuffed animals if you were performing the role of Vampirella.

Chapter 6 gave you a number of ideas for songs to match specific roles and routines. If there is a song that you feel especially confident dancing to or that has special significance for the two of you, then plan your role, costume, routine, and decor around it.

Three or four songs should be enough for your dance performance. (You'll read more on that in Chapter 9.) But your evening is hours long. Think about what you will be doing before your dance and after. Program the right music for those occasions, too. Make a tape or burn a CD or just load up the CD player, making note of the song lengths if coordination with events is important. You may have to bring the boom box along or install a speaker in another room if events are to move from one location to another.

Props work with the music and lighting to create a mood. Imagine that you are creating a scene in a romance novel. Subtle lighting and the use of mirrors will add excitement to your performance, not to mention give your partner a great view from all angles. If your event is not a surprise and you have his cooperation, blindfold your man and lead him into the room. This should increase the dramatic impact of the elaborate setting you have created.

Food

No matter where you choose to perform your seduction, if you plan to use food as part of the evening, you will probably find it easier to dispense with the cutlery and go with easy-to-eat finger foods. Put everything on one platter so that you don't have to get up and move around from whatever position you are in. Check with your local caterer. They may even have suggestions for a platter that fits your theme.

Finger foods have a built-in decadence factor. For example, for dessert, you can feed each other sensuous chocolate-coated strawberries. If you have a small fondue pot handy, you can drip the hot chocolate on each other and lick it off. (But be careful and make sure the chocolate isn't too hot.) If that isn't enough to get you going, scientific research has shown that chocolate may be the only food with aphrodisiacal qualities. One major manufacturer of perfume has already taken advantage of this fact and included chocolate as an ingredient in a scent it claims can drive men wild. All I know is I like chocolate in any form.

Alcohol may get rid of inhibitions, but contrary to popular belief, it is not an aphrodisiac. It depresses the nervous system and I don't recommend it for anyone who will be performing the moves described in this book. Nevertheless, champagne is so strongly associated with romance in our culture that some people claim it actually works as an aid to seduction.

Some foods, by virtue of their texture and temperature, have erotic connotations. Food that you can suck or roll around on your tongue gets more than your gastric juices working. Squishy edibles like gelatin can be suggestive. Warm foods are more erotic than cold foods because they are the same temperature as your body. But remember, chewy or crunchy snacks will never be erotic, even if they don't stick to your teeth or leave crumbs in your bed.

With these facts in mind, here are some favorites. Foie gras pâté is extremely erotic and can produce a significant reaction in members of the opposite sex. One gentleman I know claims that the soft and mushy texture of foie gras pâté in his mouth is the next best thing to having oral sex. If that is not to your liking, oysters also have a suggestive texture and can be used to the same effect. Beluga caviar is considered a sensual treat when entertaining.

When I was a young girl, my grandmother would force me to eat a concoction made from egg yolks, sugar, and Marsala wine. This was supposed to give me energy and strengthen my blood (or so I was told). I took it like a medicine—with great reluctance. I have since learned that it is called zabaglione (Zah-bahl-YOH-nay) in Italian (I believe we more often use the French word sabayon), and when whipped and heated in a double boiler, it becomes a sensual sauce that can be relied upon to add an erotic ambiance to intimate occasions. Like crème anglaise, it can be eaten as a luxurious stand-alone dessert or, like whipped cream, served with your favorite fruit or poured over a piece of cake.

Break the Bedroom Habit

Plan for the fact that your seductive dance may have immediate amorous consequences. Believe it or not, many couples have never had sex outside of their bedroom! (Of course, I know this isn't you.) The bedroom may turn out to be the best spot for your seduction for other reasons, but try to break old habits if you can. This seductive occasion is supposed to be different, remember? For example, if you are surprising your partner for his birthday and have a cake and dinner set up in the kitchen, why not finish the seduction right there (maybe even mixing you *and* the cake for dessert) rather than going off to the bedroom to make love after dinner?

Wherever you live, you have more than one room to choose from. There's the great outdoors, too. If you live apart from your partner, you have his place to consider as well. Suggestions for equipping other rooms and off-site locations for your passion pit will follow in this chapter.

Space is the first thing you should consider. Any room you choose should have enough floor space for you to do the moves you will be learning without knocking over any furniture. I would look for about thirty-five square feet, in addition to the space that will be occupied by his seat. Move the furniture when you create your dance floor. Take a look at the floor surface. Carpet will make your floor show more comfortable but could make some moves more difficult if you're planning to wear high heels. Like the professional strippers onstage, if you will be on a noncarpeted floor, you can always pull out your floor-show blanket for that portion of your dance.

Arrange your Lover's Throne and the other furniture so that you have lots of room to maneuver, and your lover has an unimpeded view. Make sure nothing will be in the way of your movement. Your first performance will take a lot of confidence and concentration, and you don't need to worry about knocking over the life-size Chewbacca figure he had to buy at the *Star Wars* convention last year, or have the distraction of a lamp cord crossing the carpet.

Location, Location

Decorating your seduction room may turn out to be as much fun as putting together your costume. Have some fun and be creative with whatever is available to you. If you are lacking a special prop or piece, do what you did for your costume: Check out the local second-hand store. Your partner will appreciate the effort you put in, especially if he knows you didn't spend a lot of money. Anything is possible, from a Victorian boudoir to a space station. Your imagination is the only real limit. Remember what the real-estate agent told you when you bought your home—"Location, location." It could be just as true for your seduction scene. The following are some brief examples of seduction settings created in rooms other than the bedroom.

THE BATHROOM

With their long vanities, double sinks, sunken tubs, whirlpool baths, separate stand-up shower in a separate closetlike room, many bathrooms these days are larger than spare bedrooms. If you've got a bathroom like this, you've got a passion pit! For starters, the bathroom already has a throne. Cover the toilet with a blanket and cushions to make it more comfortable for your king.

Cover the bathroom ceiling with helium-filled balloons, concentrating on the tub area. Select several colors and tie them with long ribbons. The colors of the balloons should reflect the bathroom colors so that it doesn't look like the setting for a two-year-old's birthday bash. You can have your entire meal in the bathroom, too.

Prepare the bathwater with your favorite bath oil or bubble bath. Make it hot—you won't be getting in right away. Do your striptease as a way of getting yourself into the tub. As you disrobe, toss your clothes into the tub—with attitude!

THE GARAGE

We all know how most men feel about their garages. The garage may be the only room in the house they feel is their territory alone. Add in an old car, a boat, or a motorcycle to work on and most men are happy campers. What better place could there be for the pleasure of a seduction? Make him an even happier camper when you camp out in the backseat of his SUV or Mercury Street Rod for a few hours. There should be no problem getting the floor space you need for your dance if you think ahead and move the second vehicle or the bicycles and riding mower out beforehand.

If you and your partner did a lot of your necking on car dates to get away from your parents, this may be the perfect way to rekindle some nostalgia along with the romance. Seduction in the garage is the perfect way to hang on to that lawn mower, enjoy a cold beer, and not actually have to do any chores, if you know what I mean.

LIVING ROOM

If you don't have a large bathroom, you can create the same ambiance in your living room (or any other room) by purchasing a kiddie pool. Yes, I said a kiddie pool—a two-man kiddie pool. Let the child in you come out to play. I cannot stress this enough. HAVE FUN! Put the kiddie pool in the middle of the floor. Move all your houseplants around the pool and decorate to suit your show. This may be a great way to tie your set into a routine with a South Seas or beach/surfing theme. I can hear the Hawaiian music or the Beach Boys now.

Let this be that great getaway vacation you don't have the time or money to take. Bring the vacation home to you. After your dance of seduction, the two of you can jump in the pool to cool off, or maybe to heat up. And forget about getting water on the carpet. You were just about to have it shampooed, anyway. (If you are really worried, surround the pool with colorful beach towels.) If you have a fireplace, all the better. Light a fire, even if it's summer, and have a barbecue Hawaiian-style, or at least toast some marshmallows.

Now that you've gotten out of the bedroom so to speak, maybe it's time to get out of the house. Not all possible seduction locations are to be found in the safety of your home. Privacy will be a consideration for some of these outside locations. Many couples are excited by the chance, however slim, of being caught.

Timing may also be a greater issue with any outside location if you have to lure him there for a surprise. With proper planning these risks can be kept to a minimum. Let's start with the most obvious off-site location for a seduction.

HOTEL/MOTEL ROOMS

Hotel or motel rooms have one big advantage over your own house: With a rented room you can make a mess and not have to worry about cleaning it up. In addition, upscale hotels have many features you may not have at home, such as well-appointed rooms with fabulous views, large bathrooms with sunken tubs and whirlpool jets, and large comfy beds that you don't have to make in the morning. Room service can supply any food you want so you can feel truly pampered.

There are a couple of small disadvantages to taking your activities off-site, however. For one thing, you will have to remember to bring all your supplies with you. Make a checklist ahead of time to avoid any last-minute stress. Include all the pieces to your outfit, your music and your own CD or tape player (hotels don't always supply stereos), any candles (plus matches) and props that will be used in your routine, as well as your makeup, perfume, and toiletries. You'll be making at least two trips between the room and the car.

If this is a surprise performance, you will have to check in ahead of when your partner's expected and bring your bag of goodies with you. Allow time to get everything in place and working; maybe even fit in a quick practice. You will also need an excuse to get him to the hotel and to your room. Good luck. Reward him by opening your door in your costume and watch the look on his face to see how long it takes him to clue in. No one has ever given him a surprise party like this!

THE OFFICE

If your partner has a private office, you have a location for a seduction. To pull this off, you may need to enlist the assistance of his secretary and to know the daily routines of the people who work there. If you feel comfortable, let his secretary know exactly what you are up to so that he or she can act as gatekeeper and cancel any lunchtime or after-work appointments and take any calls to ensure total privacy once you have locked the door behind you. You may need his secretary's help to get him out of the office so that you can set up the CD or tape player and close the blinds and take care of anything else you need to do to set the stage. You may also want to bring a light picnic lunch or evening snack for the two of you. To avoid the problem of changing into your costume, wear it under your coat or suit. Maybe you can dress up like a secretary or businesswoman (see Chapter 12, "How to Do Your Own Strip-A-Gram"). While the real secretary is keeping watch, you can thrill your man inside the office, just like in a movie scene!

THE BEACH

Turn a simple walk on the beach into a stripping scene. If you own resort property or vacation in one spot regularly, you probably know a secluded spot or time on a beach nearby. As you walk you can enter the water while removing articles of clothing in a sexy fashion. Discard them without care in the sand or water. This is a good opportunity to showcase that new swimsuit you would never wear to a public pool. And don't worry about losing what you are wearing—your clothes will wash back up on the shore.

Music will have to be optional. He may be already carrying the picnic basket, so asking him to carry a CD player, too, might be pushing things. And if you've never brought a stereo along to the beach before, he is bound to be suspicious or reluctant. If you've driven to your location, then use the car sound system. The farther out to sea you go, the less clothing you should have on, and the only music you will need to hear is the sound of the waves washing your clothes up on the beach. You won't have the controlled environment that you can create at home, so be prepared to improvise. What matters is *how* you take your clothes off. Keep your eyes fixed on his and smile wider with every article of clothing you remove. He won't believe you have never done this before.

There is only one more thing to add to whatever scene you have set—you! As great as your set decoration is, as seductive as your costume may be, only you can provide the sex appeal. The moves that will make your partner putty in your hands are the subject of the next three chapters.

The Basic Moves

The two things most people know **9** about strippers or exotic dancers are (a) most, if not all, of their clothes drop to the stage in the course of a performance, and (b) their bodies move in ways that other women can only dream about. Well, dream no more. These moves are simple to learn with a little practice, and have been "road-tested" in the field on countless male subjects. Arousing yourself as well as your lover is the goal. As in all things, practice  will improve your skills and confidence. You want your performance to seem smooth and effortless so that all minds (and bodies) can focus on the task at hand—getting turned on!

Since most of you won't have the space in your house or the cash in your home-renovations bank account to install a runway and pole (not to mention the problem of explaining their presence to your house guests ☺), I have collected these basic moves largely from the repertoires of professional lap and table dancers. These moves are performed by exotic dancers on or very near to their patrons, and so are the most relevant to our cause. Remember, we are engaging in a contact sport here, not a concert hall performance. The advanced moves you'll learn in the next chapter come from stage shows but are not too athletic to be beyond a woman in average shape. Learning the moves that drive men wild is the part of my workshop that women anticipate the most. I'm sure you will get a kick out of them, too.

If you can, practice in the room that will be the scene of your seduction. If not, find a place that provides equal dancing space and a similar floor surface.

☺ I know of one former showgirl who had a pole installed in her basement rec room in order to keep in shape for the occasional performance. Only her closest friends know that she ever was a dancer. She explains to guests that when the ceiling was replaced some of the joists were found to be sagging and a steel beam and pole were put in for structural reasons. I've never heard anyone question her. I don't know what she plans to tell them about the mirrors!

Be sure to practice in the outfit you will be wearing for your performance as soon as possible. You will want to be thoroughly comfortable in it come seduction night. As you shall see, your outfit will be incorporated into many of your moves. Also, for reasons of familiarity, practice with the music you have selected. It is an indispensable part of your show and will help put you in the right mood while rehearsing.

As I explained in the first chapter, my students practice their moves on Bob, my poseable and infinitely patient dummy. In your case, unless you can get the paperboy to volunteer, you will have to practice with a chair alone. Try to find one that doesn't sit too low, preferably with arms that will be sturdy enough to hold the weight of both you and your partner. This is the chair that you will use as your King's Throne as well.

The fourteen moves described on the following pages form the basic routine that I teach in my workshops. They are all you need for a complete seductive performance. The next chapter outlines ten additional moves I teach to the students who take my "advanced classes." Remember that there is no right or wrong way to do these moves. I offer them as suggestions, not set choreography. Treat them as a starting point and customize them as the spirit moves you. Like your outfit, your moves should work with your body. A comfortable fit with your personality is the only way to ensure that your natural sensuality shines through. Keep the goal of seduction uppermost in your mind. Remember, if your dancing turns you on, it will turn him on, too!

Don't overwhelm yourself by trying to put together an entire routine during your first practice. Work on each move individually until it comes naturally. No doubt ideas for combining the moves will occur as you progress. Your costume and music will also give you inspiration. I recommend choosing three songs for a total length of approximately ten minutes. (See Chapter 8, "Setting the Stage.")

As you develop your routine, you will have to start tailoring your moves to fit the length of the individual songs. As a beginner, you shouldn't try to wing this— you don't want to be left with your behind in his face and no music to shake it to! Transitions between songs will require some planning, so you will need to know exactly where they occur in your performance. When the breaks between songs come, you should be in a relaxed position, such as sitting on his lap, kneeling on the floor between his legs, or facing him with some body contact. The pause will give you a chance to focus on your next series of moves, or pull out any props you intend to use.

Q: Is a ten-minute routine enough to get a man
turned on?
A: Try ONE minute. Your biggest challenge will be to
keep him in his seat!

The following sample routine assumes you'll be wearing a costume of bra, panties or G-string, garter belt and stockings, heels, and a jacket or blouse. As Chapters 6 and 7 showed you, there are many more possibilities. A little imagination will be all you need to adapt these moves to your personal seduction-wear. As with any physical exercise program, before starting with the moves, it is best to warm up. I lead my classes through a series of simple bends and stretches. Use whatever routine you feel comfortable with.

1. The Strut and Snuggle

I have said it before in this book, but nowhere does it apply more than when performing your seduction dance: ATTITUDE IS EVERYTHING. The first move to master is walking with attitude—the strut. This will put you in the right frame of mind for your whole performance.

The best way to put attitude into your walk is to borrow the visualization technique used by actors. Here's what works for me. As I enter the room, I imagine that I am a millionaire walking into a bank. In my purse is a million dollars. The banking staff, knowing this, hold their breath and direct me to the manager. He is overly grateful and polite as he receives my money for investment. When he invests it, instantaneously I receive another million dollars as a return on my initial investment. When I walk out of that bank, I imagine I'm a million dollars richer *just like that!* Now, *that's* attitude!

Strutting involves your whole body. With your head held high, set your hair in motion by moving your head or by fluffing it with your fingers. Hold on to the front of your jacket, blouse, or sweater right at the level of, and on either side of, your breasts. I like to start my strut wearing a jacket or blazer because of the wonderful opportunities for showy movement it provides. With your hands outside your jacket or top, walk around the room and manipulate and rotate your breasts in slow, loving motions. Snuggle them as though they are your most treasured possessions. Recall the warmth and secure feeling of your softest flannel pajamas on your bare skin. Show your pleasure in every gesture you make and every look on your face. As you move about the room in time to the music, maintain eye contact with the occupant of the Throne, and let him know that all your sexy feelings are directed toward him.

2. Adjust Your Partner's Legs

When you arrive at the Throne, your partner may have his legs closed or crossed. Make him comfortable by gently lifting the crossed leg and placing it on the floor. Spread his legs to allow enough room for you to fit in between them. If his arms are crossed, place his open hands palms down on the arms of the chair, or on his thighs. A relaxed pose will put him in a more receptive frame of mind. You should be standing close but not too close just yet. Once he is comfortable, you will begin to relax yourself. Your job is about to get more fun.

Make any leg adjustments part of your performance. While you adjust him, bend over with a naughty look on your face, and keep your eyes on him. Eye contact is always desirable. With a long, sultry stare, place your hands just above his knees and give his legs a little squeeze. Now you are both ready for move #3.

3. Stirring the Pot

Stirring the Pot is a classic and essential move in the repertoire of any exotic dancer. It involves the broad swiveling of your hips and can be used in conjunction with many of the other moves you will soon learn. Practice it until it becomes second nature. When all else fails, or you forget what to do, you can always stir the pot. It's like having a foolproof recipe. The name *Stirring the Pot* is a clue to the way the move is performed. Start once you have adjusted your partner's legs and are standing just out of reach but directly in front of him.

Have you ever cooked a pot of chili? If not, you have likely eaten it at some point. Maybe chicken soup? Okay, everyone has made chicken soup, if only out of the can. The difference between the two is very noticeable. Chili contains many heavy ingredients, such as ground meat, beans, and onions, and tends to thicken as it cooks. When stirring its contents, you need to scrape the sides of the pot to keep the chili from sticking. Chicken soup, on the other hand, contains fewer ingredients and consists mostly of water. With chicken soup, you can get away with just sloshing it around a little without actually stirring all the way around the sides of the pot.

To stir the pot, think of your body as a long spoon. Move your hips in a counterclockwise, circular motion as if stirring with them, and *think chicken soup*. Keep your right foot slightly ahead of your left foot and your hands touching your body, maybe on your knees. Gently slosh that chicken soup around, keeping your knees slightly bent to permit greater movement at your hips. Your knees will be tracing a small circle, too, and permitting gentle up-and-down motions in your upper body. When you can do all this smoothly and comfortably, you know you are stirring the pot. If you really want to draw attention to the seductive power of your hips, *think chili*. Use all the same movements, but make them slower, more deliberate, and increase the diameter of your circular motion to scrape the sides of the pot. Throughout your performance, you will be adding other moves on top of this one, so it is important that you get it down pat. Most of the time, this move will be all you will need. If you forget what to do, simply stir the pot.

4. Stir the Pot and Turn

Place your left foot in the center of an imaginary circle and your right foot about eight inches in front and to the right. Your right foot will trace the outside of the circle and lead you around in a counterclockwise direction. Pivot from toe to heel alternating from your right foot to your left foot, lifting your feet off the ground ever so slightly as you turn. Remember that your hips are stirring the pot in a counterclockwise direction the whole time your body is turning. Keep your hands on your hips as you turn and stop when you have your back to your partner.

By the time you are done, you will never look at

cooking the same way again. A silly grin will be on your face every time you put that wooden spoon into a pot. Martha Stewart should have it so good. I wonder what she thinks about when she stirs her pot?

When performing these dance moves, keep some space between you and the Throne. A few men, even in these circumstances, don't like their personal space to be invaded. Likely, you are already aware of how your man is regarding this point. Keep in mind, too, as we've said before, that men are highly visual creatures. More than us, they are turned on by what they see. Your man will want a full view of your body as you dance provocatively in front of him. Gauge your distance according to your height: Tall women should be farther back than short women. Keeping your distance will also keep you away from his clutching hands. (It may seem as though he has about five of them.)

5. Off with the Jacket

Facing away from your partner, grasp your jacket or blouse at your breasts and spread your arms out as far as the jacket or blouse will allow. Keep your head held high and your back arched. Wiggle your jacket or blouse from side to side, sliding it off your shoulders. Then let go of the jacket and drop your arms to your sides and shimmy your shoulders until the jacket falls to your waist. Bend forward and pull your arms out of the sleeves. Your butt should be sticking out all the way, forming a ledge, and your upper body should be parallel to the floor. Your jacket or blouse will rest on your hips and cover your extended butt. You are now in position for the Queen's Wave.

6. Queen's Wave

Queen Elizabeth has a wave that is recognized all over the world. With your newfound attitude, you are the Queen of your own domain, and will need your own distinctive wave. Unlike the British monarch, though, you won't be sending a message with your hand.

Leave your top where it is and remain in your bent-forward position. Place your hands on your knees for support and arch your back with your butt pointing in the direction of your loyal subject. Working from your hips, trace a sideways figure eight with your bottom: top left to bottom right; up; top right to bottom left; and up to the top left. Repeat as necessary. It's just like waves in the ocean. Since you have your back to your partner, be sure to look over your shoulder with an expression that sends your message home.

7. Jacket Toss

Okay, so now your butt is waving like the Queen and is covered up by your jacket or blouse. Time to get rid of that! Still with your upper body parallel to the floor, move your butt to the right, keeping your left hand on your hip. Use your right hand to grab your jacket or blouse and slowly pull it off, exposing your behind. Return to the vertical position and resume stirring the pot. Swing your jacket or blouse slowly over your head in a full circle and let it land on your right shoulder. Keep stirring the pot and turning until you are facing your partner. With a look that says "I'm in control here," toss your jacket or blouse wherever you want it to go. Now your attitude is showing! One down and lots more to go.

8. Boobs on Bob

As you stand in front of your partner, play with your breasts. Your jacket or blouse is off now and your bra is exposed. Fondle your breasts with your eyes closed. Really enjoy your own body for a moment or two before you continue. Make sure his legs are spread just wide enough to allow room for your body. Facing him, allow your hands to trace down your body and on down to your knees.

Move your hands from your knees over to his. Trace up from his knees until your hands are on his thighs. Shift your weight onto your arms and keep your legs straight as you gently lean into his body. Your breasts should be touching his chest as you stare lovingly into his eyes.

9. Front Slide

With your boobs now on *your* Bob, you are ready to begin the Front Slide. Start your *slooooow* slide down. Hold his gaze as long as you can, and maintain frontal contact at all times. As you glide down, tracing his body with your hands, bend your knees until you are kneeling on the floor between his legs. Your breasts should now be in his lap. Trace your hands down his legs to his ankles. It will take a bit of practice to get the distances and timing right so that you end up in the correct position. Once you have, look up into his eyes with a fabulous smile on your face. Let him know that you actually meant to wind up on the floor. Yes, between his legs is exactly where you want to be.

10. Getting Up

Now that you're on the floor, how do you get up? With grace and ease, of course. As you recall, your hands are touching your partner's ankles. Move them over to your knees and trace your own body all the way up to your breasts. Holding your breasts, lean forward toward his crotch. Place your hands on his thighs and use the strength in your arms to pull you off the ground. Don't squeeze too hard. As you come up, keep your head down and pull away from his body, letting your hands find your legs. Trace them up your body. Once again, practice will be necessary to make this move appear smooth and sexy. Return to stirring the pot and turn again (see #4) until your back is to your partner.

11. Dropping Your Skirt

With your hands on your hips, trace your body gracefully with your fingertips all the way down to your ankles. Practice this move over and over until you can do it with poise. At first it will look like you are trying to keep your balance. When you reach your ankles, you can peek at your partner between your legs before you trace your body on the way back up.

If your zipper is on the right, stick your hip out to the right like you did just before you took your top off, and slowly undo your zipper, stirring the pot in time to the music. Tracing your body again, hook your fingers inside the waistband of your skirt. This time as you slide your hands down your body, take your skirt with you. When you get it down to your ankles, gently move it away from your feet. Trace your hands back up to your hips, and lift your right foot out of the circle formed by your skirt. Your legs will now be slightly spread. Use your left foot to catch hold of your skirt and toss it out of the way. Once again, do it with attitude! Stir the pot, turn, and face your partner.

12. Leg Up

If you are wearing a garter and stockings, here is your opportunity to show off your luscious lower limbs. Move to a position between your partner's legs, gently lift your right leg, and place your foot just above his left knee. Be gentle as you place your foot there, and avoid stabbing his leg with your high heels.

As you show off your leg, look him directly in the eyes. Trace your hand slowly down from your hip, covering the entire length of your leg. Start again by tracing the shape of your butt as you turn it slightly to face him. Have your hand go to the back garter-belt hook. You can give it a gentle tug or a snap before actually undoing it. Leave the front garter done up so that he suffers in anticipation. Let the garter dangle as you place that leg back down and repeat the process for the other leg.

Funny, but the more clothes you remove, the hotter it gets in the room.

13. Boob and Hair Play

Stir the pot some more as you move your hands away from the garter belt and up your body. Play with your boobs as if you just grew them today. The look on your face will demonstrate just how wonderful it feels to have a pair of hands touching your boobs. He will agree. Be gentle and manipulate them slowly without pausing. Remember, his hands are living vicariously through yours.

Gradually let your hands move away from your boobs. Make him wonder what your hands will do next. Tracing with your fingers, move your hands up your chest, along your shoulders, and up your neck. Circle around to the back of your neck and start playing with your hair. Fluff it out gently as you tilt your head from side to side. Run your fingers through your hair and treat yourself to a gentle scalp massage. I like to close my eyes halfway and pretend I am at the hairdresser's for a wash and massage. Please don't stop. A little moan wouldn't hurt right about now. Ohhhhh . . . that feels soooo goood.

14. Emptying Your Cups

Okay, so you have already removed your jacket and skirt and undone one garter on each leg. You can stop here if you want to keep him guessing (or start your messing) *or* you can proceed to free yourself of bra and panties. Yes? Okay, here we go . . .

Stir the pot and turn the way you learned in steps #3 and #4. Keep on doing so until you are facing your partner. Now do the Boobs on Bob and the Front Slide, only this time when you find yourself on your knees in front of your Bob, you can reach around (if it is a back latch) and undo your bra. Don't let the bra fall just yet. Slip one strap at a time off your shoulders and cross your arms in front of your breasts as if you're trying to hide them. Lovingly remove your bra and toss it on top of your mounting clothing pile.

If you are feeling especially playful, gently place the cups of the bra over his eyes like a blindfold and hook it up behind his head so it stays on his face. Or if the spirit moves you further, stand up, strut around behind the Throne, and gently tip his head back. Place your boobs one on each eye. As you pull away, a gentle kiss on the forehead will let him know you are doing this as a labor of love (or a must for lust).

Advanced Moves

For many of you, a

10

performance incorporating the first

fourteen moves will be all you need to get

your partner's blood and other bodily

fluids percolating. But as with coffee,

someone always wants a stronger cup. For

those people, I have included ten

additional moves that I teach my graduates

in our master class. Unlike the first

fourteen moves, they don't go together in

the order I have listed them to make a

routine. Use them wherever

they fit into the routine you

are creating. But exercise

caution: These moves are more athletic and not intended for people with back problems. If you perfect any of these moves and use them in your performance, your partner will certainly sense the time and effort you have put into improving your love life. He may want to enroll in a fitness program just to keep up! Or, as in the case of one of my students, he may even let you go pro.

This particular student—let's call her Sally—showed a great deal of natural attitude and learned the basic moves easily. She had an open, fun, and loving relationship with Ed, who waited eagerly at home to be teased and played with. It wasn't long before he got his wish. He, too, noticed her ability and commented that she was good enough to do it professionally. That set Sally's wheels in motion.

Sally and Ed had three children at home. Sally hadn't worked since the second one came along and money was a little tight. What household couldn't use a little extra money? The two of them headed for a club I suggested and started their research. They both sat and watched the dancers on several different nights so Sally would feel comfortable. Sally returned with a friend of hers, another student of mine, to further study the dancers' moves and note the music they chose to dance to. She also talked to the disk jockey and got as much information from him as she could.

Finally Sally gathered up her nerve, made arrangements to perform, called her friend to join her, and headed for the club. Remembering what she had learned about attitude and confidence, she strutted her stuff. The club patrons, she learned, could be as nervous as she was. The first night was profitable. Ed didn't mind the baby-sitting and was more than happy to help her practice for "work." Everybody benefited from the extra money coming in, and Ed rather enjoyed the idea that his wife was so attractive to other men.

1. Dirty Dancing

Here is a move you can try while you are down there between your man's legs, facing him on the floor. Rub your boobs in his crotch for a while, dirty-dancing style. Then hold on to his thighs and pull yourself up. As you rise, throw your legs one by one over his so that you are straddling him and looking into his face. Feel free to give him a kiss or two if the mood strikes you, or run your fingers through his hair. Lean up against him with your boobs in solid contact and start undressing him little by little as passion demands. Just when he thinks he's about to strike oil, slide off his lap and stir the pot some more. Somebody has to do the cooking or you would both starve.

2. G-string Fling

Now that your bra is a mere memory, all that re-
mains is your panties or G-string. (High heels don't
count. No man ever wants you to take them off!) Time
to repeat the Front Slide. This time your breasts are
bare, so be careful you don't scratch yourself on any buttons or pant zippers your partner may still have closed.
When your knees touch the floor, swing your legs to the
right and sit back on your left butt cheek. Lean backward on your elbows and stretch your legs out in front
of you, keeping them together as you raise them in the
air. Point your toes and do circular motions by rotating
your legs from your knees, which should be bent. Next,
stop rotating your legs but keep them in the air and your
toes pointed upward as you lie on your back. Wriggle
your butt back and forth as you free your panties or
G-string from under you. Slide them all the way up
your legs until they reach your ankles. Now take your
right foot and bend it toward you until your heel is
pointing straight up. Lift the right panty leg opening
over your toe and hook it onto the heel of your right
shoe as you slide your left foot out of the left panty leg
opening. Point the heel of your right shoe at your target,
stretch the panty back like a slingshot as far as it will go,
and send your panties—and your partner—to the moon!

3. Stocking Stretch

Some women like the look of garters and stockings so much they leave them on for their entire routine . . . and beyond. Removing them, however, provides wonderful erotic possibilities.

If you are following move #12, Leg Up, from the last chapter, your back garter will already be dangling; now it's time to undo the front one. While sitting on your partner's lap, lean over to one side and turn your head back to look at him.

Make a statement by snapping your garter boldly before undoing it to let him know it's *almost* time. With the garter undone, tuck one finger from each hand under the top band of the stocking on each side of your thigh and gently start tracing your leg down to your ankle, taking the stocking with you. Slip your heel out of your shoe, being careful to keep it balanced on your big toe, and then toss it onto the top of the pile of clothes. Slip the stocking over your ankle and along your foot until you can pinch it between your big and second toes. Holding the stocking tightly between your toes, stretch it out, *allllllll the wayyyyyyyy*. Play with it and have fun. Put the thigh part in your mouth and chew on it. Make hand-job gestures with your hand around the stocking. When you have had enough, you can fling it away or wrap it around his neck and gently pull him toward you.

These last moves illustrate a very important point to keep in mind as you create your performance. By all means, practice, practice, practice, but remember to stay flexible. Making the moves second nature will give you the confidence and skill to improvise should you ever have to. And you will. Even the best-laid plans can go awry. Keeping a sense of fun will help get you through those moments. The G-string as slingshot came about as a result of one of those moments.

One day while doing a floor show, I removed my G-string as I had many times before. Only this time when I slid it down my leg, the elastic strap accidentally hooked on the heel of my shoe. I decided to stay on the floor and leave it there. Playing with it for a while, I teased the audience by threatening to fling it at them. A few of the patrons in the front row picked up on the joke and ducked to avoid getting hit in the eye. When my G-string finally did take flight, it landed with a splash right in a pitcher of beer. The guy who owned the pitcher calmly reached in, plucked out the G-string, wrung it out into the pitcher, and proceeded to pour himself a glass of the freshly squeezed brew. The crowd roared with laughter. His buddies all wanted a glass. I crawled on all fours over to where they were sitting and, with the tips of my index and forefingers, claimed my beer-drenched undies. My look of disgust and disbelief soon turned to laughter as I appreciated the humor of the situation, and the audacity of this patron. From that time on, the G-string Fling became a part of my routine. My aim improved, too. Whenever I was faced with a rowdy crowd, I would aim for their heads, or, if possible, their crotches. Even when I missed, the trick was a hit.

4. Lap Dance Bump and Grind

Begin by stirring the pot and playing with your boobs as you turn. When your back is facing your partner, trace your body down to your knees and bend forward. Then reach backward with your hands until you can feel your partner's knees. You need to know where they are because you will be straightening up to sit on them without looking back. Push his knees closer together if necessary to form a lap. Still facing away from him, carefully sit on your partner's lap and lean backward toward one of his shoulders. (You don't want to bang his face with your head.) Like a sex kitten just out of her cage, you could suck on your fingers or chew on the tip of his tie. Try pointing the tip of your tongue and flicking it back and forth as you turn your head to gaze into his eyes. (You might want to practice this beforehand in front of a mirror when no one is around. It can be very sexy when done well.) Settling deeper into his lap, bump and grind while you arch your back and roll your shoulders. You should be able to feel, literally, your partner's passion. Don't grind so hard that you could hurt him. You will know how much pressure to apply. Let your butt cheeks be your (and his) guide.

5. Back Slide

Now that you've been in his lap, you should really have him going. Use your hands to play with your boobs and leave your hands there as you tuck your elbows against your sides. Then position your elbows on his legs and lower yourself to the floor. As with the Front Slide, you will be between his legs, but instead you'll be facing out. As you lower yourself down, spread your legs until they are in a wide V-shape by the time your butt touches down. You are now ready for the Scissors.

6. Scissors

The Scissors is one of those moves that put "exotic" in exotic dancing. If he hasn't figured it out by now, he'll know you have had professional instruction when he sees this move.

Your partner is now looking down at you from his chair while you are sitting on the floor between his legs. Start with your head back and nestled in his crotch and looking up into his eyes. Since you've just finished the Back Slide, your hands will still be holding your boobs. Take them off your boobs and place them on the floor slightly behind your butt. Use them to push your lower body forward a few inches. Point your toes and put both legs together as though closing a pair of scissors. Now bend your right knee upward and cross it over your left leg. Let your right leg lead your whole body around until you are kneeling on the floor facing the Throne. With your right knee still bent, you are ready to start crawling on the floor.

7. Cat Crawl

Now you are ready to start purring. With practice, you should be able to move across the floor with feline grace. The Cat Crawl isn't designed to cover large distances, so don't worry that your room might be too small.

First, get on all fours and spin your entire body around on your right knee until you are pointing away from your partner. With your hands directly underneath your shoulders and your knees only six inches apart, slide your left knee forward until it touches the heel of your left hand. At the same time, extend your right leg backward until your leg is straight. Your left knee will be touching the floor and taking enough weight to allow you to slide your right hand forward six inches. Now, bring your right knee forward to your right hand while extending your left leg backward and sliding your left hand forward. Repeating these movements several times will move your body forward in small baby steps.

The way your butt moves as you crawl away will mesmerize your partner. He may make some distinctly inhuman sounds himself by now and wish to join in. Studying Eartha Kitt in an old *Batman* episode may give you some pointers on feline sensuality. Who doesn't want to pet a cute kitty?

8. Everyone Gets Up

Meeooow, how do I get up now? It's easy! Spin around to face him, and crawl like the cat you are over to his feet. Get in close enough to trace his legs all the way up to his knees. By the time you have done this, you are up on your knees, too. Now trace a little further up to his thighs and pull yourself up onto your feet using the strength in your arms. Keeping your head down, trace your hands back toward his knees. While you're at it, you can unzip any zippers, unbutton any buttons, or rearrange any shirttails that need rearranging. Who knows what a curious cat might find in there? Finally, move your hands to your own knees. Trace your body gracefully up toward your boobs as you straighten up, then toss your mane back—with cattitude!

9. Fun with Props

With a bit of preplanning, props can be introduced into your performance. There are lots of possibilities here; let your imagination run free. Here are a couple ideas:

Start by sitting on the floor and leaning back on your elbows, facing your partner. Spread your legs in the air (with or without your G-string on) and reach over next to you for an ice cube from a bowl you've placed ahead of time on the floor. He should be able to see your face framed between your legs. Put an ice cube in your mouth and slosh it around until it starts to melt. Take the melting cube out of your mouth and rub it on your chest and nipples, then use it to trace your body down to your belly button. Next, swing both your legs around and onto the floor on one side so that your hip is up and your butt is facing him, then trace the cube down to your butt. Squeeze the cheeks of your butt several times—now you're winking at him! (Don't forget that whenever your legs are up in the air, your toes should be pointed.)

Even when you were a child, you knew that whipped cream had more pleasure potential than just eating it could provide. Even if he isn't known for his sweet tooth, your man is sure to go for this classic. Put whipped cream on your nipples, belly button, and pubic area. Make sure you explore the theatrical possibilities of the spray can and its foamy contents. Crawl over to your partner, grab him by the tie, and let him enjoy his dessert. No thought of calories tonight!

If you plan to use any additional toppings out of your refrigerator, think about possible stains and take reasonable precautions. But try not to worry about explaining to your housekeeper how you got blueberry stains on your satin panties. She's seen it all before, and you don't owe her any explanations. A little pre-wash soaking is a small price to pay for a carefree night of fun and frolic.

10. The Chair Show

Here is a chance to be sexy and give your feet a bit of a rest from all the work they've been doing in high heels. Choose a sturdy wooden chair with arms and place it off to the side before you begin your routine. A faux fur blanket or thin cushion will ease the pressure on your butt for the next set of moves.

Strut across the room and with one hand grab the back of your chair. Lean it toward you so that the two back legs are dragging on the ground as you pull it to the perfect viewing spot three or four feet in front of and facing the Throne. Trace the back of the chair with your fingers just before you move around in front of it. Stir the pot as you turn your back to your partner and then place both hands on the seat of the chair. Stick your butt out and do the Queen's Wave. Stir the pot some more and turn slowly to face your partner.

Run your hands down to your knees, letting your head hang down. As you straighten up, toss your hair back and move your hands behind you to locate the chair. Ease yourself into the seat and rotate until you are sideways in the chair. Lean back and play with your breasts and slide your butt to the edge of the seat. Lift your legs and point your toes as you make circular motions with your legs.

This may be a good time to slip your panties off. Slide them all the way up to your ankles while you stare straight into his eyes. Slip one foot out and hook the other opening on to your other foot. Fling your panties with an attitude of wild abandon. For an alternative, try kneeling on the chair with your back to your partner. Arch your back as far as you dare while doing a grind with your butt. Tip your head back and let your hair hang down, baby. (Like I said, these moves are not for people with back problems.)

The chair show has a lot of potential you may wish to explore. Anything done in a chair looks hot when done well. He'll never know you're using it to get off your feet. So have a seat, relax, and play with yourself for a while. He'll love to watch!

Up Close and Personal

You've just devoted a lot of time **11**
to deciding on your role, your costume,
and the theme and decor for your evening
of seduction. Your head is probably still
spinning with the number and variety of
moves that are possible. But there is still
one more lesson to learn: *You must make*
your partner feel that he is an active
participant in his own seduction. This
might be a little easier if he has been aware
of your plans. But even then, you will have
been careful not to let him
know exactly what to expect
when you are finally alone

together, so an element of surprise will be a part of every seduction, and with it the risk of making him feel awkward or uncomfortable.

The way to avoid this, besides being confident and relaxed yourself, is to sprinkle your performance with a number of simple gestures that add a personal, more intimate flavor to your seduction. For the purposes of this chapter I am assuming that you will be incorporating these gestures into your dance routine wherever appropriate, perhaps even in time to the music, and that your partner is sitting upright in his Throne. But there is no reason you can't use one or more of these gestures to fill a few moments between songs. Heck, there is no reason you can't use them at any time in a playful loving relationship—so long as no one is looking!

Removing His Tie

Removing a man's tie is a simple task if your only intent is to get it off his neck and out of the way. But if your intention is seduction, there are a few things you need to know.

Start by sitting sideways on your partner's lap with both your legs to the left and lean slightly backward and to the right. Gaze into his eyes as you reach out with your right hand and pick up his tie at its tip. Slide it over your left shoulder as you ease gently off his lap to a kneeling position facing him between his legs. Leave the tie knotted for now. Place the tip between your front teeth and, as you pull it taut, begin stroking it. Your motions will look like you are reeling in a rope, but you won't actually be pulling on the tie. Your motions will also look like something else he will recognize. Let out a little growl between your clenched teeth. He should be getting the message loud and clear by now.

On your last stroke, lean your body closely into his crotch and grind. Reach up to the knot in his tie and gently undo it. Be sure to unbutton any button-down collars. Once the tie is untied, repeat your stroking motions. This time you actually will be grasping the tie and pulling it from around his neck. Do so slowly and in short motions to avoid strangling him, and continue until the tie is completely off and lying in his lap. Lean your face into his crotch, pick the tie up with your teeth, and toss it out of the way with a flick of your head. A purr or a growl will convey your attitude.

Undoing His Shirt

Is he wearing a jacket? If he hasn't taken that off himself by now, give him some assistance from behind the chair. If he has been grabby and too eager to get to the horizontal part of the evening, leave his jacket on for now. Pull the shoulders down around his elbows, making a straitjacket of sorts. You can still undo a few shirt buttons with him in this position if he promises to behave. Make him sit and take it until you are good and ready to release his restless arms.

Start by standing in front of your partner and between his legs. Beginning at the top of his shirt, undo one button at a time until you get down to his waist. Unfasten any buttons at his sleeves. Then untuck his shirt slowly with seductive flare, one side at a time. Unfasten the top of his pants if that is necessary to release the shirt, then undo any remaining lower shirt buttons. Move your hands around his waist to his back, untucking as you go. Maintain eye contact as much as possible. It should always look like you are concentrating on him and not on what you are doing. That is the mark of a real pro. Leave the shirt on until the room gets even hotter.

Removing a Belt

This can be just as sexy as removing his tie, and you can use his belt to show him who is boss when he misbehaves. Start by straddling his lap and sitting so that you face him. Kiss his neck or let your hair fall in his face, giving him a good whiff of your perfume. As you look directly into his eyes, unbuckle his belt. Once the buckle is undone, you can slide off his lap in a Front Slide, keeping your chest in contact with his body, especially when you reach his crotch area. Then, with your head close to his crotch, grasp the buckle end of the belt and *slooooowly* pull it from his pants. As you pull, stroke the belt as if it were his favorite toy. Take your time, and look at him, not at the belt. When you have pulled the belt out from the loops, hold the end without the buckle in front of your mouth. Lick your lips and flick your tongue. (See Tongue Curl, below.) This action will give him a hint of pleasures to come.

Once you are done "eating" the belt, you can take it with one hand on each end and loop it over his head. Then insert the end of the belt into the buckle and tighten it up around his neck, pulling him ever so gently toward you for a little kiss on the lips. You're

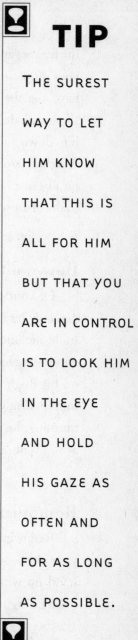

TIP

THE SUREST WAY TO LET HIM KNOW THAT THIS IS ALL FOR HIM BUT THAT YOU ARE IN CONTROL IS TO LOOK HIM IN THE EYE AND HOLD HIS GAZE AS OFTEN AND FOR AS LONG AS POSSIBLE.

the teacher and this is Domination 101. Pull him toward your nipple so he can say hello. Or, if he promises to behave, use the belt to pull him onto the dance floor for a slow, sexy dance. If he's one of your better students, sit him down and release your grip on the belt, but leave it dangling around his neck until class is dismissed. If he's been a bad boy, sit him back down and tie him up to the chair with the belt.

Beware the Garter Snake

Of course, if you are feeling overworked, you can certainly let him lend you a helping hand. If your costume includes them, those troublesome garters are a good place for him to start. While you have your leg up on his thigh, point your finger to the garter hook and motion firmly for some action. Like a boy on Christmas morning, he will be all thumbs and boundless enthusiasm. Eventually he will figure it out and unclip it.

Removing Your Glove

Removing a glove can be as enticing as removing your skirt—with a little help from him. Hold your left hand up with your elbow bent at a right angle, your palm facing toward you, and your index finger pointing to heaven. With your right hand, begin unrolling your glove slowly upward from your elbow. When you get to your wrist, place your index finger between your front teeth and, with your lips parted, shake your head back and forth playfully as you pull the glove off your finger. Repeat with the next three fingers. Place the last finger of your glove in his mouth and let him know you would welcome a little help from his clenched teeth. With a look of approval, slowly pull your hand out of your glove. A little tug of war is always fun. Give in and let him have it!

The Art of Touch

Most of the moves you learned in Chapters 9 and 10 are done tantalizingly out of his reach or right in his face. This is surely what the "tease" in striptease is all about. But there is also a middle ground where erotic expectations are enhanced through artful touching. The following moves can be integrated into your performance or used on a date or on any occasion when you want to win more than just his heart. Even if someone else is watching, he'll know that the message you're sending is for him only.

Dancing around behind him, run your fingers through his hair, and maybe rub his temples with a few brief strokes. Lick his ears or give him a little kiss on the neck or cheek. Doing this from behind heightens the erotic effect by adding an element of surprise.

Dancing around in front of him, accidentally drop something so you can bend over. Allow him that illicit peek up your skirt. Stand up and turn around slowly to give him a chance to pretend he wasn't looking. The same effect can be achieved as you face him by reaching for something in such a way as to expose the bounty of your cleavage. In either event, maintain your air of superiority with a sly look that says, "I'll decide what you see and when you see it, so don't play games with me." Oh, you're both playing games all right. Only this one has two winners.

As you dance around behind him, give your man's shoulders a gentle squeeze. If the occasion allows, extend your attention to a thirty-second massage to loosen the tension in his shoulders and increase the tension in his lower brain. Still behind him, run your hands and arms down his chest, pausing to undo any buttons that might still be fastened. Slide your hands into his shirt and feel the exposed skin on his chest. Give him goose bumps as you trace his skin with your fingernails. Let your hand continue its travels outside his shirt and down to where it can accidentally brush against that bulge in his pants. Ooops, you don't want to give him too much too soon. Tease, tease, tease, and more tease!

Hair Toss

Long, wavy, blond, curly, black—whatever your style and color, men just love hair. Use every opportunity available to let it touch his bare skin wherever that occurs. With one hand, start at your shoulder and slowly trace your fingers up your neck toward your ear and run your fingers through your hair. As you trace your hand back down your neck, fling your hair around and let it graze his face. Fluff it up with both hands like the girls in the conditioner commercials and put a sexy pout on your lips.

Tongue Curl

Back when we thought a tongue was for licking Popsicles, we would get a swat if we stuck it out in someone's direction. Now we realize what a wonderful erotic tool a tongue can be in the extended position. You may want to practice this in front of a mirror. With your mouth open wide, stick your tongue out and down as far as it will go. No, further than that. Now point and flick the tip up and down. Use your newfound talent on the tips of ties, the ends of belts, your own stockings, and any other tools at hand.

SEDUCING A

MAN IS LIKE

RAISING A

CHILD:

YOU MUST

GIVE HIM

EVERYTHING

HE NEEDS

BUT NOT

EVERYTHING

HE WANTS.

Butt Slap

Butt slapping has been around since mastodon was haute cuisine. Who knows why it works, but it speaks to the caveman in every man. Facing away from your partner, arch your butt out to the right and put your right hand on your right hip. Glance over your shoulder at your partner with your naughtiest look and then gently give yourself a little swat on your behind with your open hand. Doing it in slow motion looks especially attractive. You're a *baaaad* girl.

A male friend of mine has seen professional strippers on many occasions and even paid for a lap dance or two. So having a woman get in close and do her stuff is not new territory to him. Yet when someone he knew well (not someone from a class of mine) tried to do a dance for him once, he felt embarrassment, not arousal. She was trying too hard without knowing what she was doing. He felt uncomfortable just sitting there waiting through some awkward pauses and not knowing how to react.

When I asked for specifics, he came to the conclusion that the problem was her failure to involve *him* in the seduction. My friend might as well have been Bob the Dummy. She didn't take his hands—or put the brakes to his hands—or touch him in any way other than to climb on him as though he were a piece of furniture. Worst of all, she never looked him in the eyes. So there is a lesson here: Above all, your seduction must be about *him*. Then the sex that follows will be about *you*.

You have had a lot of information to absorb so far, and naturally you will be devoting a lot of your concentration just to the movements that are new to you. Don't hesitate to practice, practice, practice—even the simplest things, such as those that form the content of this chapter. You want the techniques of seduction to be a part of your character, a natural expression of your inner feelings, and not an act you adopt for a special occasion. Your partner has one big asset going for him that my friend didn't enjoy, and that's your deep and long-standing feelings for him. Let those feelings guide you in your seduction.

How to Do Your Own Strip-A-Gram

It was lunchtime, so Sherri waited in Mr. Bryant's plush inner office for him to return from his meeting with other insurance industry executives. It was very important to create the right impression, so she had taken great care to dress that morning. Sherri was wearing her favorite little navy suit with white pinstripes and white cuffs and collar. The skirt went to just below the knee and the closely fitted jacket was cinched in by a one-inch-wide navy belt. With her hair all tied up in a bun on her head, a red scarf tied around her neck, and glasses, Sherri looked every inch the prim secretary.

"There's a rather bold woman here to see you, Mr. Bryant," she heard his secretary tell him as he arrived in the outer office. "No, she doesn't have an appointment, and I don't know what she wants."

A man of about sixty-five years of age walked in. Mr. Bryant was wearing a conservative suit and tie and a puzzled, perhaps somewhat annoyed look on his face. Sherri introduced herself and told him she had some very important business to discuss with him. Holding Mr. Bryant's attention, Sherri moved over to the tape player she had placed out of sight and pushed Play. Out blasted Dolly Parton's song "9 to 5."

This was just the signal the staff had been waiting for. Barely stifling their giggles, a crowd gathered in Mr. Bryant's doorway and outer office. He knew he had been had, but could see no escape route when Sherri started into her routine. When he retreated to the chair behind his desk, she pulled him back out where everyone could see and sat in his lap to take dictation. Always the pro, Sherri danced around for the entire song, in and out of his lap, removing only her little necktie, which she tucked into his lapel pocket. With a grand movement, Sherri let her hair down and tossed it in his face. It was hard working nine to five!

"She works hard for the money," sang Donna Summer as Sherri *slooowwwllllly* undid all the buttons on the front of her jacket. By the end of the song, her hands had moved around to the zipper on the back of her skirt and Johnny Paycheck began shouting, "Take this job and shove it!" That was Sherri's cue to drop her skirt to the floor, bend down provocatively, and . . . shove it. She picked the skirt up and tossed it into Mr. Bryant's lap. By this time, his face matched the color of Sherri's scarf in his pocket.

The fourth and last song Sherri had chosen was appropriately titled "I'm Out of Work." The men in the office were very attentive as her lace teddy gave way to bra and thong panties. But the women seemed to enjoy the whole experience more than the men. Their eyes got bigger and bigger the more clothes Sherri removed. Stripping was all new for them. Perhaps they enjoyed seeing the boss so uncomfortable, so not in control. When it was over, Sherri slowly undid Mr. Bryant's fly, bent down between his legs, and left a big red lipstick mark on his Fruit of the Looms. The onlookers thought he was going to have a heart attack. Oh my God, he must have been thinking—how was he going to explain to his wife that lipstick prints on his shorts were just a retirement gift from a thankful staff?

Perhaps you don't live with your partner. Maybe it

is very difficult to get privacy where either of you live because of families. Or maybe you just don't have enough room. "Strip-a-grams" like the one described above are the perfect solution for the woman who lives apart from her man, or the woman who wants to surprise him at his office or somewhere else outside his home. Take a look at what you have learned so far. Why hire a pro when you now have the skills and confidence to do a strip-a-gram yourself?

Sherri's secretary show was the obvious choice for the businessman about to retire. There are many more occasions when a Hallmark card is not enough—only a strip-a-gram will do. Coming up with an idea for your strip-a-gram can be a lot of fun. Is your partner's birthday approaching? Do you celebrate the day you met each other? Your wedding anniversary? How about honoring the time you first got naked together? Every couple has their own private anniversaries to celebrate. The strip-a-gram should be something that you *both* enjoy. Take a look back at some of the performance ideas described in Chapter 6 and see if you find something you can adapt for your purposes.

In Chapter 5 we talked about scheduling your seduction scene for a time when your partner would be most receptive. That applies doubly to a strip-a-gram. It is important that your strip-a-gram performance be

TIP

THE SURPRISE ELEMENT OF A STRIP-A-GRAM IS OVER QUICKLY. BEST KEEP YOUR PERFORMANCE UNDER TEN MINUTES. THREE OR FOUR SHORT SONGS ARE THE MOST YOU WILL NEED.

tailored to the time of day and occasion. For example, you don't want to be a dominatrix for a lunchtime surprise if somebody at work has already been dominating him all morning!

Any wild or upbeat role makes more sense at night, when everyone has left work behind and wound down a little. Subtle humor works best during the daytime. A clown or the little girl with her lollipops (see Chapter 6) are two routines that I would suggest. Think about it. A clown with her balloons or a cute little girl bearing sweet treats can get into a workplace or private occasion without letting doormen or receptionists know what is really about to happen behind closed doors!

A dancer and former *Penthouse* cover model and centerfold I know, who calls herself Molly O, quit dancing in May 1984 to raise her children. But Molly O soon found that while you can take the dancer out of the show, you can't take the show out of the dancer. When she returned to the profession,

Molly learned that exotic dancing had changed since she had left, and she liked performing onstage too much to be a lap or table dancer. Her solution was to perform strip-a-grams. Since hooking up with an agency, Molly O has done shows for every occasion and every kind of person imaginable. Her surprised clients have been young men turning eighteen, retirees at sixty-five, the infirm and disabled, men who were celebrating birthdays, divorces, promotions, stags, etc.

Make My Day

Molly's favorite and best-received show is her Cop Show. Her policewoman's uniform includes *everything* but the arm badges. Any well-planned strip-a-gram is going to be a surprise, of course, but the way Molly and the agency manager Walter plan it, the surprise goes beyond a pleasant moment of confusion and sudden realization. No, what Molly's victims have in store are a few long minutes of off-the-scale stress followed by the near collapse of relief.

Walter frequently drives Molly to the stags to ensure her safety. On one occasion the two were sitting outside in the car, keeping a low profile and waiting for just the right time for Molly to make her entrance. Inside was the usual scene at a stag—drinking, gambling, and a few porno movies on the screen. As Molly and Walter waited, the groom casually walked outside and smoked a joint with the best man in his car, only one spot over in the parking lot. Molly and Walter tried to be inconspicuous as they slid down in the front seat.

Shortly after the two smokers had moved back inside, the best man returned to give the signal to Molly. Unknown to the groom, he was in on the scheme. Molly made no secret of her entrance as she strutted around the room in full uniform—including billy stick and handcuffs. Finding the groom, she announced that she had been in an unmarked car and had just seen him smoking marijuana outside. The groom's once happy face now registered horror. What's more, Molly stated that she had found something in the front seat after a quick search. Holding up a bag that only she, Walter, and the best man knew contained oregano, she informed the groom that he was under arrest. He turned white as a ghost and offered no resistance as she proceeded to handcuff him.

The groom was speechless and mortified as Molly escorted him to a cleared area in the middle of the room and handcuffed him to a chair. Meanwhile, Walter had slid over to an electrical outlet and plugged in the stereo. Everyone but the groom was laughing by the time Madonna could be heard singing "This is a bust." When

Molly began to dance and strip, the groom finally started to relax, although he'd sure straightened out in a hurry, and his buzz was totally gone.

Molly has another routine that works especially well in the corporate world, a place where propriety is on everyone's mind. Perfectly groomed and attired in a business suit, Molly appears in the victim's office pretending to be looking for a job. She gives the boss a real sob story, telling him she is willing to do anything to get the job—*anything,* you understand—because she really needs the money. Wink, wink. Of course, the interviewer finds this highly unusual, but her straight face tells him that maybe she is telling the truth. Her body tells him this is an offer he should consider. He blushes a bit when she tells him how good-looking he is. Now he knows something is not right. Or maybe it is right. His ego kicks in and he's snared in the trap. The rest of the scene proceeds much like Sherri's secretary scenario described at the beginning of this chapter. The psychological trap placed at the beginning makes Molly's strip-a-grams unique. Molly likes that sinister element and all the planning and research that go into her "stings."

Here's a funny strip-a-gram of Molly's that would be a good one for a first-timer to try. Molly shows up at a birthday party dressed in regular party clothes and begins mingling with the guests. The person who hired her quietly puts the word out to the bartender and all the guests not to let her drink too much because she has a reputation for getting out of hand. Naturally, the men start buying her drinks, hoping for exactly that outcome. When no one's looking, Molly disposes of the drinks, but the party guests still see what they expect to see—a woman staggering around and leaning on men, talking and laughing too loud, generally losing control as she becomes increasingly intoxicated. Just as she has everyone's attention, she grabs the birthday boy, and with the carefully selected birthday music cued up, proceeds to do a special dance just for him. When the party guests see her move like a pro with lots of attitude, they laugh with relief and enjoy the show.

If you have come this far in the book, chances are you enjoy the rush you get from adopting a new character and planning and executing a big surprise. Add in the feeling of power one gets from controlling a seduction scene and you've got an intoxicating mix many women can't resist. If that sounds like you, the strip-a-gram may be your best weapon. Use some of Molly's great scenarios as the inspiration to let your imagination run wild! At least it's still legal. So choose a couple of songs, put your fur coat over that lace teddy, slip into your best heels, knock on his door, and dance your heart out. Get ready to knock your partner's socks off!

Do It Just Because

It was a beautiful day in the **13** early summer and the seven of us had no trouble agreeing to dine at a trendy outdoor café downtown. My companions were all women with many successes in their personal and business lives. Our conversation started with an update on one another and what we were doing to keep busy, and drifted, as these gab fests inevitably do, to our relationships with the men in our lives. As the cocktails took hold, there was a lot of frank talk and a lot of laughter. Getting up to leave, one woman who had been leading much of the conversation announced, "I'm sorry ladies, but I must go home and perform my wifely duties."

I didn't laugh with the others. It was a joke, of course, but judging from her previous comments that evening, it masked a truth. My first reaction was disgust. Later, after I had time to reflect, I became dismayed and saddened. How tragic it was for both her and her husband that she viewed lovemaking as a major chore. Was it because sex had become routine and boring for her? Or, more serious, was it because she viewed lovemaking as something she must do for her husband in order to get the things in life that could truly make her happy?

The women who attend my workshops have already decided to take responsibility for their relationships and to improve them by learning to strip for their partners. I am aware, however, that some women—not the ones who take my workshops—view my activities in a negative light. They see my lessons as encouraging women to accept a subordinate role. Learning to strip for a man could only mean you are trying to earn his favor, they would say. No doubt the woman described above would hold this view.

Nothing could be further from the truth.

Yes, seduce your man, but *do it for yourself!* And do it just because. Take the lessons this book has to offer and make romance, and maybe even a little seduction, a part of the way you live your life every day. Say good-bye to bedtime boredom and romantic routine.

Just Because

Some of us may have been in the same relationships for a long time. We sometimes take our partners for granted and they do the same with us. Hanging around the house in sweatpants and sweatshirt seems like a comfortable thing to do every day. After all, who is going to see you there? Only your partner, and you're not worried about what he thinks. He's been with you all these years. He's not going anywhere, you're thinking—he's probably as comfortable with you as you are with him, right? Wrong!

Being comfortable with his circumstances doesn't mean he won't accept an improvement. He'll welcome your seduction with open eyes *and* pants. But don't drop your seduction—or yourself—in his lap all at once. Remember that you live with someone who sees you every day of the week, day in and day out, for better or worse. A sudden shift to the passionate vixen one night might leave him startled and confused. Get out of your rut *now* and start doing special and effortless little things every day that will kindle a spark in your relationship and prepare both of you for the passionate nights you have planned.

Little by little, start doing things you don't usually do—things like setting a beautiful table for dinner in the middle of the week for no reason. And hold no expectations. Often, when women prepare a fabulous meal and set an inviting table, men look at them like something is going on. What does she want? they think. Well, don't want anything. Simply do it just because. And then keep doing little things like that several times a week. This is the "random acts of kindness" school of thinking applied to your domestic life.

Perhaps you don't go to bed in your special lingerie except on those nights when you desire sex (or, heaven forbid, something else). Well, go to bed in your special lingerie any day of the week—just because. Don't do it because you want sex or anything else. Do it just to pamper yourself. If you usually wear your pajamas until noon on Saturday, put on a nice casual dress after you take your morning shower—just because. If you never wear makeup at home, start flattering your natural good looks with some new cosmetics and wear your hair in an attractive new way—just because. Not for him, for yourself.

You'll be amazed at how your life will change around you. At first your partner may wonder what's up, even if he knows you are planning a seduction for him. But eventually when he adjusts to the random acts of kindness you have injected into his life and learns that you have no direct expectations as a result of your actions, he will come around. I don't believe any man can't be changed in the light of this new approach on your part. Watch him start to do more things for you around the house. I'm betting his appearance will start improving, too. He'll be standing up straighter and sucking in his gut with a smile on his face, and all this without nagging from you! At first he may have wondered if you were having an affair. Now he knows the answer is yes—and he's the other man!

I am fully aware that many of the women who join my workshops do not actually do a seductive dance for their partners. But that doesn't mean they are getting nothing from the class. On the contrary, they consistently and emphatically report an improvement in their self-esteem and confidence. Here are a few examples from my former students:

"I feel a million times better about myself, and know that if I really wanted to, I now have the tools and ability to do a striptease for my partner," one woman reports.

"[Mary's workshop] helped me to be more confident, something I was not taught growing up," reports another.

One woman felt so good, she volunteered to be in my next demonstration video. Another, as we learned earlier in this book, became a professional stripper.

Overcoming the fear of stripping for someone else

is the push that first gets this self-esteem/self-confidence ball rolling. From there, many things become possible. One woman told me my workshop helped her to overcome her shyness. Once she allowed herself to be so self-expressed in front of the class with no negative consequences, she realized she had nothing left to fear and became more outgoing. She didn't have a partner at the time, but I'll bet she has one now.

Along with their self-confidence, the women I instruct describe a new acceptance of their bodies and a deeper understanding of their sensuality:

"I have overcome my inhibitions about my body and feel very comfortable, especially when I start to play with myself," one woman told me.

From another: "The best idea I got was to develop my sexuality and playfulness."

"I now have more confidence in myself and my body," is a typical comment.

Most women are excited by all the things they learn in the workshop. Initially they think they are there to learn a few sexy moves to use at home or on the dance floor. They end up doing a lot more erotic movement than they anticipated. They are pleasantly surprised when they discover role-playing and the possibilities it opens up for costume creation and set decoration. Until they took the workshop, they assumed there was only one or two sexy ways to dress or act. The seduction experience stimulates their overall creativity and gives them a chance to express their femininity and have fun at the same time.

I'm All for Play

I never hear this directly from my students, but I have become aware of another more concrete benefit arising from doing a striptease for your partner. The women I met in the café at the beginning of this chapter touched on this subject as we laughed and talked. Although their sex lives could be satisfying on the whole, they complained that they didn't get enough foreplay before making love. "As soon as I take my clothes off, he's in there wanting to have sex right away." Sound familiar? Stripping is the ultimate form of foreplay. And as any experienced seductress will tell you, when you do the stripping, you are in control. So much for the "subordinate role" theory. Review all the moves and gestures you have learned from this book with foreplay in mind. Notice how many opportunities there are to initiate and control the pace of foreplay?

Think of yourself as a teacher. Having a penis doesn't make your man an expert on foreplay any more than having a womb makes you an excellent mother.

You had to learn about your own sensuality yourself. And you just learned more by reading this book. So have patience and learn about what turns both of you on—together.

Maybe I should have called this book *Stripping: The Ultimate Form of Foreplay*. Along with the more intangible benefits noted above, that is really what it has been about, hasn't it? And that's perfectly fine. Foreplay reminds us of our humanity. Note that the word ends in *play*. Playing is what children do naturally, and what we adults forget how to do. Because playing is spontaneous and unconscious, it is a pure expression of joy. And Lord knows we could all use a bit more of that in our lives.

Our first romances were pure expressions of joy. Despite our inexperience and naïveté, it all came so naturally and with a powerful intensity, didn't it? I believe that unconsciously we all seek the same high we got from that first love throughout our lives. That is why you are holding this book in your hands right now. We both know you won't get your first love back, but you could very well get the feeling back. And what is more important, with all the things you have learned, your current love can be your last love. Good luck.

Contact Information

Mary Taylor
Live Girl Productions Inc.
Website: www.peelandplay.com
E-mail: mtaylor@peelandplay.com

Toll free phone number: 1-888-295-PEEL (7335)

Video: *Art of Seduction: How to Strip for Your Partner*
CD: *Sounds of Seduction*
Book: *Bedroom Games*
Workshops: "Peel and Play" Workshops
Speaking Engagements: "The Art of Seduction"

About the Author

By the age of nineteen, Mary Taylor was a divorced single mother who needed a better way to provide for herself and her child than her low-paying part-time job as a medical receptionist. But nothing in her traditional Catholic, Italian-immigrant background had prepared her for the career she would soon adopt. A chance encounter brought her to the office of veteran stripper Lori Lane, who soon persuaded Mary that her youthful beauty could more than quadruple her current earnings. The adrenaline high of Mary's first performance and a standing ovation from an enthusiastic audience got her hooked, and a lucrative new career was born.

Throughout the seventies and eighties, the exotic dancing industry changed rapidly, and the glamour and excitement that first drew Mary in was disappearing. Feature dancers were the last reminders of a colorful burlesque past, and they had to travel farther and farther from home to earn a living. Table dancing, and later lap dancing, had changed exotic dancing from stage play to little more than foreplay. Finally, after twenty-one years, Mary quit dancing.

Faced with the same challenge she had faced as a nineteen-year-old single mother, Mary again searched for a new career path. But what do twenty-one years spent as a stripper prepare you to do?

Teach others to strip, that's what! With a lot of hard work (and the steadfast assistance of Bob the Dummy) Mary created her "Peel and Play" workshops. Soon women everywhere were seeking her professional help and learning to overcome their fears, gain self-confidence, and fan the embers of their love lives into raging fires.

Mary's *Art of Seduction* video and *Sounds of Seduction* CD soon brought her lessons to a wider audience. Now *Bedroom Games* makes her inspirational message and sure-fire seductive techniques available to every woman in North America. Our love lives will never be the same!

Mary continues to be active as an advocate for the rights of exotic dancers as she works with local agencies to improve dancers' frequently miserable working conditions. Her "Peel and Play" workshops and public speaking engagements are growing more popular and attracting increasing attention from the public and the media.

Mary lives in the countryside outside Toronto, Ontario, with her German shepherd.

Peel and Play Journal

Use these blank pages to record your thoughts, feelings, and ideas about *Bedroom Games* . . . and enjoy your newly invigorated love life!